The Skin Whisperer

A DERMATOLOGIST REVEALS HOW TO LOOK YOUNGER, RADIATE BEAUTY AND LIVE THE LIFE YOU CRAVE

By KEIRA L. BARR, MD

The ideas discussed within this book are based solely on the opinions of Dr. Keira L. Barr, based on her years of study, her practice of dermatology and her personal experience, and may not reflect every doctor's perspective. The information and material provided within this book are for educational purposes only and the content is not intended to replace the advice of your dermatologist, physician or health care provider. Before you make major dietary changes, start an exercise routine or begin a skincare regimen, it is important that you consult with your physician regarding the safety and applicability of the information contained herein to your unique and specific concerns, symptoms or condition. Following any of the recommendations in this book does not constitute a doctor-patient relationship. The intent of the author is only to offer information to help you in your journey towards improved health and emotional wellbeing. Use of any information in this book is with the understanding that the author and publisher expressly disclaim any responsibility for any adverse effects arising from the use or application of the content contained herein.

Copyright © 2018 by KEIRA L. Barr, MD

All rights reserved. No part of this publication may be reproduced, distributed, or transmitted in any form or by any means, including photocopying, recording, or other electronic or mechanical methods, without the prior written permission of the author except in the case of brief quotations embodied in critical reviews and certain other non-commercial uses permitted by copyright law. For permission requests, write to the author, addressed "Attention: Permissions Coordinator," at the email address below.

The Skin Whisperer: A Dermatologist Reveals How to Look Younger, Radiate Beauty and Live the Life You Crave

1st Edition. 2018

ISBN 13: 978-1986036856
ISBN 10: 1986036855

CONTACT THE AUTHOR
Business Name: RESILIENT HEALTH INSTITUTE
Main Website: www.drkeirabarr.com
LinkedIn: https://linkedin.com/in/keirabarr
Facebook: https://www.facebook.com/resiliencyblueprint/
Book Bonus: https://www.drskinwhisperer.com
Email: drbarr@chooseresilience.com

Table of Contents

ACKNOWLEDGEMENTS v
PREFACE vii
INTRODUCTION xi
TAKE NOTICE 1
THE SKIN YOU'RE IN 9
WHY SPF ISN'T YOUR ONLY BFF 35
NOURISH INSIDE OUT AND OUTSIDE IN 59
BEAUTY SLEEP IS REAL 123
STRESS PERCEPTION 135
ART OF COMMUNICATION 141
SELF-CARE IS NOT SELFISH 151
FINAL THOUGHTS 163

REFERENCES 165
ABOUT THE AUTHOR 179

ACKNOWLEDGEMENTS

To the one who has always seen, heard and supported me every step of the way and championed me when I was not yet ready to do it for myself. An inspiration and beacon of light to everyone he meets, my best friend, my husband. I am the luckiest gal in the world to have you by my side.

To my children, who amaze me on a daily basis with their curiosity, tenacity and resilience, who inspire me and make me so incredibly proud. The traits they possess I had not fully realized at their ages. Self-image and the stories that narrate our personal, professional and spiritual choices are created when we are young. Unless we can awaken our senses and write our stories in alignment with our passions and our purpose, we cannot fully thrive. Kelen and Cole are already well on their way to writing their own lives and thriving. They are the reason I'm compelled to share my message.

To my parents and sister for their unconditional love, support and guidance. My gratitude and love has no bounds.

To my amazing colleagues, mentors, clients and friends. I feel so fortunate to have crossed paths and am grateful for all that you have given and that we have shared.

And to those of you reading this book, the ones I have the joy of knowing personally and those I have not yet had the pleasure. I am honored that you are sharing your time with me as you read these pages. You are my big why. It is a privilege to serve and support you as you embark on your journey towards personal and professional discovery, growth and transformation.

PREFACE

The Skin Whisperer is the culmination of over 20 years of training, experience and wisdom sown by working with amazing patients, colleagues and mentors. It is also the product of a lifetime of self-discovery.

This is not your typical dermatology text. As such, allow me to take a moment to share with you what to expect as you read this book.

First of all, *The Skin Whisperer* book is not intended to be a guide about what lotions, potions and products to use on your skin. My mission is to help you build the strongest possible foundation upon which your overall health and wellbeing will flourish. The products you use on the surface of your skin will have little impact if you do not address all aspects of nourishing and nurturing what lies beneath it. Rest assured, if you need recommendations after reading this book, I've got you covered, but within these pages I have intentionally left out such product suggestions.

Most importantly, this book is designed to engage you in the act of better looking after and learning about your skin. Throughout the book, there are opportunities for you to dive deeper into the topics we cover, as well as getting more educational material whenever you need further information.

Mostly, this book is intended for your contemplation and understanding of skin and the way you treat yours. Throughout it, I invite you to take notice of what you are currently doing and help you explore changes that are possible. In *The Skin Whisperer* book, I provide knowledge to help you to make informed choices and empower you towards greater skin health transformation. Developing an awareness of how you are living creates opportunities to pursue what you want, what you crave, and what ignites your passion and purpose.

The information in this book is not a quick fix. There are ideas, suggestions and concepts that you can implement if you choose, but making any sort of change takes time, patience, practice and commitment. The old adage of it being a "marathon not a sprint" applies to what you will find in these pages as well. Give yourself permission to soak up what you can, when you can, and circle back as many times as you need.

People differ on the length of time it takes to establish a habit. For some, it's 21 days, others 90 days, and many require even longer. No matter what it is for you, it's okay. The only request I make is that you don't give up completely. You're reading this book because you are committed to your health and wellbeing. Remember, you are amazing, and amazing creations require nourishment and nurturing in order to thrive. And thriving takes time!

Lastly, this book is an opportunity for us to get to know each other, start a conversation, establish trust, create a bond and open the door to deepening this work together in the future.

PREFACE

Having been on this journey myself, I want to help make it easier for you by offering support, guidance and knowledge to add value to your life and the lives you touch.

As you enjoy the book, if it resonates with you, I'd love to hear from you and learn how I can further support you. The best way to reach me is by visiting www.drkeirabarr.com or sending a note to drbarr@chooseresilience.com

By visiting the link in the box below, you can gain access to additional resources, and learn more about how you can look younger, radiate beauty and live the life you crave.

I look forward to embarking on this journey with you!

With big love and gratitude,

Dr. Keira

Here are you resources:

www.drskinwhisperer.com

INTRODUCTION

"With realization of one's own potential and self-confidence in one's ability, one can build a better world."

Dalai Lama

I believe everyone deserves to feel comfortable in their skin and I believe that potential exists inside of each one of us.

Feeling comfortable is not just about what's **on** our skin; it's also what's happening **beneath** it. I can relate to feeling uncomfortable in both.

Even though I'm now a skincare expert as a dermatologist, my youth and young adulthood was spent worshipping the sun, trying to mask the shame and embarrassment of how uncomfortable I felt with who I was in my skin. As a child, kids at school made fun of the two birthmarks on my face and called me Coffee Stain Face. In those moments, I became acutely aware that my skin could be a source of pain, shame and humiliation. I soon figured out that if I got a tan, my "coffee stains" became less noticeable, almost invisible, so I took every opportunity I could to keep them that way.

As the daughter of a redhead, I have fair skin with a tendency to burn but I ignored this warning sign. Years of subjecting my skin to sunburns and suntans led to sun damage, freckles, and moles. It culminated in diagnosing myself with the most deadly skin cancer there is: melanoma.

When I saw that spot on my arm, my heart sank and panic set it in. I knew that something was seriously not right. This particular mole had been on my arm for years, but on that day when I checked my skin, it looked different… darker… more irregular in contour. I was scared and that fear was compounded by the fact I had the skills to interpret the findings microscopically. I could see the features of skin cancer clearly right in front of me. There was no denying it and my colleagues agreed. Waves of nausea mixed with disbelief washed over me. As a dermatologist, I became my own worst nightmare patient.

If I'd known then what I know now, I wouldn't have had the shock and upset of finding that spot on my arm and had to undergo surgery. I don't want that experience for you. I never want that to happen to your children or anyone else's.

For most of my life, I carried the emotional scars from my childhood and allowed them to shape my sense of self. I allowed feelings of shame and embarrassment about what was on my skin to diminish my self-esteem and self-confidence. It was from this place of poor self-image that I chose how to nourish — or more accurately stated, starve — my skin, body, mind and soul of what it truly needed to thrive.

I, like so many women, have looked at my own reflection to find that **what** and **who** I saw in that mirror was a source of stress, anxiety and overwhelm.

INTRODUCTION

As a physician, I felt I should have known how to take care of myself. After all, I had nearly 20 years of medical training under my belt. My skin cancer diagnosis proved me wrong. At the time of my diagnosis, I felt I was "doing everything right" with regards to wearing sunscreen, keeping up with the latest trends and using the hottest new skincare products on the market, as well as getting exercise. In fact, I thought I was in the best shape of my life during this time because I was running marathons and ultra-marathons. But clearly, I was wrong.

Contrary to what I believed throughout most of my young life, my experience taught me that our skin is not the enemy; in fact, it's the hero. It protects us. It lets us know what our body truly needs to thrive.

The diagnosis of skin cancer was my wake-up call about how I was living and what I was doing. The accumulation of freckles and moles over the years was my skin's way of whispering to me, "Hey, I'm trying to protect you." The moles that started to grow and change color over the years was my skin's way of talking to me, "Hey, I'm losing ground here, I'm doing what I can but I need your help." And then finding that spot on my arm — that melanoma — was my skin shouting at me, "Hey, seriously! I'm maxed out."

Despite being a dermatologist, I hadn't been listening to what my skin had been desperately trying to communicate to me for over a decade. It took being diagnosed with melanoma to hear the message. Finally. This was the turning point for me. The reality was that things would never improve until I stopped looking for strategies to treat what was on the surface and started paying attention to what was happening beneath. In order to look younger, create lasting health and pursue what I wanted in my life, I had to uncover the truth about what my skin was telling me about my current state of health. I had to identify the issues holding me back and develop a new way of thinking about "skincare."

For what seemed like the first time, I was taking notice of how I lived my life. As I tuned in, it became clear that what was showing up on my skin was directly correlated to the choices I had been making. I realized I had to make new choices. I began to make changes in how I nourished my body nutritionally, emotionally, physically, and spiritually. It was only then that things begin to shift. I went from nearly a decade of biopsies and surgeries every few months for growing and changing skin lesions to not having to have a biopsy in the last five years because I haven't needed one.

Although a hard lesson to learn, my experience served as the catalyst that transformed my body and self-esteem, and gave me the confidence to know that I am in control of my health. I can change my habits. I can make new decisions.

You can too.

I don't want you to have to endure the same experience I did. I most certainly don't want you to be diagnosed with skin cancer. And although this book isn't about skin cancer specifically, rest assured, I am going to walk you through exactly what you need to know to protect yourself as well as what to look for.

Because I have been on this journey, I am not going to tell you or ask you do to things that I am not willing to do myself. Do I do them perfectly? Nope… because guess what. There is no perfect. It's about making progress, being consistent and forgiving yourself when you take a detour. I'm here to lay out a roadmap for you, as well as actionable steps you can take, starting today. My hope for you is that through this journey you begin to hear your body's needs when they are still just whispers, not shouting, like they were in my case.

In *The Skin Whisperer* book, I'll address how to evaluate your skin and show you how to nourish yourself, body and mind. I'll guide you to nurture those kind and caring habits so you can create the life you crave and live it. I'll share strategies rooted in science to keep you feeling younger, healthier and more confident from the inside out.

Feeling comfortable and confident in your skin is the true meaning of skincare and together we can make it your reality.

Chapter 1
TAKE NOTICE

*"It's not what you look at that matters,
it's what you see."*

Henry David Thoreau

When you look in the mirror, is the sight of new onset adult acne, mottled pigmentation and wrinkles a source of frustration or anxiety? What do you avoid in your life because of the anxiety you feel about your skin? When you see your reflection in the mirror with blemishes on your skin, what thoughts are running through your mind? Are they nurturing and supportive or are they belittling and degrading? And what if there was a simple way of alleviating the anxiety you experience on a daily basis? Just by looking? Just using your power of observation? Would you give it a try? How would that change your life? What would you do differently if you knew that nourishing your body and mind was the solution to improving your skin health and emotional wellbeing?

All this change might seem overwhelming right now, or even impossible, so let's start at the beginning — by observing and understanding a few basics about the skin you're in.

As your largest organ, your skin has many important functions. One of them is serving as a reflection of your overall state of wellbeing, which shows up on your skin in various forms. The key to understanding how to properly nourish yourself is to use your power of observation and **take notice** of what you see and the clues that may provide.

Being diagnosed with skin cancer was a pretty big clue for me that my body needed something I had not been giving it. What that something might be was not immediately apparent to me. I had been using sunscreen. I was no longer sunbathing. I was eating what I thought was "healthy" food. I was running marathons. I thought I was taking care of myself, doing everything right, but my skin was telling me otherwise and clearly letting me know something needed to change.

Dermatology is a very visual specialty, so my power of observation around what was on my skin surface was not the issue. I could readily diagnose what I saw on the skin, but the solution to making a change was using what I saw to understand *why* I was seeing it. This would require that I truly took notice… with each one of my senses.

I invite you to do the same. In the next chapter, I will lead you step by step on how to examine your skin and what to look for specifically as it pertains to skin cancer, but for now I am asking you only to **awaken your senses**. As you begin to develop an awareness of what you are seeing, feeling and experiencing on your skin, in your body and in your mind, you'll be able to use those messages to dig deeper, interpret what they could mean and take them as an opportunity or catalyst to make changes for yourself. In short, your senses can clue you in to what to do next, whether that is something you can impact yourself or even seeking the support of a medical professional.

I know it can be feel awkward. It can be tough to dig deep, but I am here for you. Throughout this book, we will address all of these issues and I will provide guidance along the way.

You are not alone.

First, I ask you that you begin to observe how you are nourishing your body, from the food you are eating to the relationship you have with that food. How are you eating? Are you eating on the go or do you take time out to sit down for a meal? Do you feel differently when you add in or exclude certain foods from your diet?

Next, start to pay attention to the products you put on your skin. Your skin serves as a protective barrier, but it is still permeable and a significant proportion of what you put on it gets absorbed. How many different personal care products do you use in a day? Hair care products, makeup, cleansers? Take notice of what you use most often.

How are you sleeping? Do you sleep like a rock or do you have challenges falling or staying asleep? Do you have a nighttime routine or do you go full speed ahead working on your computer or watching TV until you collapse into bed? Is your sleep environment like a cozy dark cave or is there bright light leaking in? What are you doing in bed before you sleep? Eating, reading, watching TV, stressing out, arguing, meditating or enjoying a satisfying romp with your partner?

Tune into the thoughts going through your mind. Can you quiet your mind on command or is there constant chatter running in the background? If there is a running dialogue, what is the tone of the conversation and what themes or topics are repeating themselves?

Take notice of how you are spending your time and with whom you are spending it. How do you feel when you are in their company? Who are you when you are with them?

Ask yourself what you do to take care of you. What activities are you regularly involved in that make you happy? What do you do that gives you meaning and fulfills your purpose? If you're not sure, ask yourself what you really want. What is it that you crave? What makes your heart race and gives you butterflies?

You can write your thoughts below or grab a journal, notebook or digital screen nearby and jot down your observations. There are no right or wrong answers, nor judgement. This exercise is simply to raise awareness and elevate your power of observation. Give yourself permission to ask yourself these questions honestly, openly and completely so you can gather as much data as possible.

As I learned from being deaf to my skin's whisper, it is only when we take notice that we can take action.

Note your observations below:

1.

2.

3.

4.

5.

6.

Now that you've made your own observations. I invite you to take it one step further and take **the Skin Whisperer quiz** to discover how your skin may be trying to talk to you right now.

Taking **the Skin Whisperer quiz** is the first step in taking notice of how in-tune you are with your skin's messages!

Directions: Tally up your score from your answers. Use your total score to discover how your skin is speaking to you and how to live the life you crave. Have fun!

1. When reaching for food, are you aware of your "why" for eating?
    - 1 (Never)
    - 2 (Rarely)
    - 3 (Sometimes)
    - 4 (Usually)
    - 5 (Almost Always)

2. When eating a meal, do you stop eating before being "stuffed"?
    - 1 (Never)
    - 2 (Rarely)
    - 3 (Sometimes)
    - 4 (Usually)
    - 5 (Almost Always)

3. In the last 6 months, how often have you engaged in activities that make you happy, give you butterflies or make your heart sing?
    - 1 (Never)
    - 2 (2-3 times)

- 3 (Once a month)
- 4 (Weekly)
- 5 (Daily)

4. How often do you listen to and follow your "gut feelings" about a decision or a person?

- 1 (Never)
- 2 (Rarely)
- 3 (Sometimes)
- 4 (Usually)
- 5 (Almost Always)

5. When you are tired do you have a nighttime routine or do you go full speed ahead working on your computer or watching TV until you collapse into bed?

- 1 (Never)
- 2 (Rarely)
- 3 (Sometimes)
- 4 (Usually)
- 5 (Almost Always)

6. Are you aware of the number and contents of products you are using on your body daily?

- 1 (Never)
- 2 (Rarely)

- 3 (Sometimes)
- 4 (Usually)
- 5 (Almost Always)

7. When you experience pain or discomfort in your joints and muscles, do you stop activities that worsen your pain?

- 1 (Never)
- 2 (Rarely)
- 3 (Sometimes)
- 4 (Usually)
- 5 (Almost Always)

Tally up your score _____

Now that you have your Skin Whisperer quiz score, find your range and discover how your skin is sending its message.

Whisper (31-35): Congratulations! You are already taking notice of the messages your body is sending you through your skin. Reading this book will help you become fluent in your skin's language and set you up for success of preventing problems before they reach the surface. You can use your power of observation to utilize all of the resources and information in these pages to create the life you crave.

Talking (24-30): If your skin is talking, reading through these chapters and doing the associated exercises will help you build the foundation of your observational powers so you can take notice and take action. Follow the recommendations to leverage your new observational skills to create radiant health and skin. You deserve to live the life you crave.

Shouting (<24): If your skin is shouting, don't panic. This is where I was too, and I'm here to support and guide you in gaining your ability to listen to the language of your skin and care for yourself. The Skin Whisperer is the perfect way for you to learn the language of your skin and begin listening to the messages your skin is sending. I will help you increase your ability to take notice and implement your skin wisdom with two simple steps: nourishing and nurturing your skin and your body. Even small improvements in your ability to understand what your skin is telling you can make a big difference in your health and happiness.

Taking care of yourself both on the surface and the person who lives beneath has incredible benefits. Increasing energy, self-esteem, self-confidence, feeling more in control of your life, overcoming feelings of anxiety and overwhelm, feeling younger, being aligned with your passion and purpose, and comfortable with what and who you see in the mirror — this is the **true definition** of skincare. With these benefits, wouldn't you want to do everything you can to take care of the skin you're in?

> **Swift Skin Action**
> Download the quiz and start taking notice of your skin.
> www.drskinwhisperer.com

Chapter 2:
THE SKIN YOU'RE IN

"Take care of your body, it is the only place you have to live."

Jim Rohn

Your skin is your largest organ, but how often do you actually think about it? Maybe you think about it all the time. Maybe you think about how it's letting you down, because you've just broken out in a huge zit right before a big event. Or perhaps your skin has this crazy rash and you have no idea where it came from, but you really want it to go away because you're going on vacation tomorrow. Or maybe you look in the mirror and you see dark circles under your eyes, fine lines, wrinkles, uneven pigmentation and "age spots", and you don't recognize the person looking back at you. I get it. I do the same thing sometimes. I look at my skin and I'm trying to figure out what's going on.

But how often do you think about your skin and the positive things that it can do for you? As your largest organ, it performs incredibly complex functions. Consider this... Your skin protects you from the outside world, guards your internal organs, plays a large role in your immune system and protects you from infection. It absorbs, secretes and excretes to keep your skin hydrated, regulate your body temperature, and detoxify waste and metabolites from your body. It not only produces hormones, but has a role to play in regulating hormones throughout your body. With so many nerve receptors in your skin, it allows you to feel. It allows you to feel the sensual, the good stuff. It also allows you to feel pain, alerting you that something isn't quite right and that you need to take action. As the initiating source of vitamin D production, your skin plays a major part in maintaining your bone health, boosting your mood and brain function, keeping your lungs and heart healthy, and decreasing your risk of cancer. And not just skin cancer, but also others, including breast and lung cancer.

Your skin, as your largest organ, is pretty amazing. Sure, you may not always like what you see on your skin, but when you see things, they're clues to something happening deeper in your body and they can give you a lot of information about what that might be. Your skin is a true window to and reflection of your overall state of health and wellbeing. And if you can tune in to what your skin is trying to tell you, you can take action to nourish it to look better, feel better and become more confident in the skin you're in.

But before you can truly understand what your skin is trying to tell you, it is important for you to understand what your skin is made of and what impacts it.

SKIN BASICS

Your skin is made up of three layers: the epidermis, the dermis, and the subcutis.

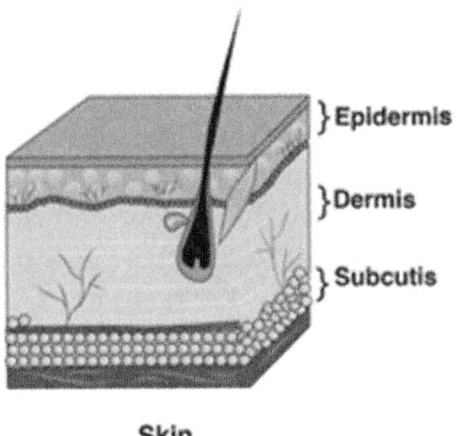

Skin

The Epidermis

There's total truth in that silly schoolyard joke: "your epidermis is showing." The epidermis is the outermost layer of your skin, and as such, is the most visible and vulnerable to irritation, inflammation, infection and signs of aging. It is thinnest on your eyelids and thickest on your palms and soles. This is important and one of the reasons why you've likely been told not to share eye makeup with your girlfriends, because your protective barrier is much thinner here and everything get absorbed more readily, including infections.

Your skin can look radiant, hydrated, plump and youthful or thin, dry and wrinkled depending on how your epidermis is doing. Approximately every month, your skin cells, known as keratinocytes, cycle from the bottom layer or basal layer, to the top layer, the stratum corneum, where they die and slough off. This process slows down with age, sun exposure and environmental toxins. This slowdown causes the layer of older cells to build up and clump, making your skin look dull, flaky, sallow and yes... older. This is why people rave about exfoliating treatments, because they make you look younger. They remove your top layer of dead skin cells and reveal your newer younger looking ones. I wish I could tell you that this cyclical replacement of your epidermal cells results in your skin being as soft, plump and pristine as a baby's bottom, but the uneven pigment and scaly patches stick around because the apparatus that creates the new cells ages and becomes impaired. But here's the good news I can tell you: the lifestyle measures I'll be sharing with you can significantly improve your skin's appearance, tone, and resilience.

What is important to know is that the most common types of skin cancer, basal cell carcinoma and squamous cell carcinoma, also known as non-melanoma skin cancer (NMSC), are made from cells in the epidermis.

Your epidermis also contains melanocytes, which are normally located in the basal layer. These are cells that create pigment called melanin that gives your skin (and hair) its color. Within the melanocytes melanin pigment is packaged into melanosomes. Racial differences in skin color are not due to differences in the number of melanocytes. Rather, it is the number, size and distribution of melanosomes or pigment granules within keratinocytes that determine skin color differences. Fair skin has fewer melanosomes and dark skin has more. Chronic sun exposure can trigger your melanocytes to produce larger melanosomes causing darkening of your skin. In other words, melanin serves as your body's natural sunscreen. Think of melanin as the ultimate accessory for your DNA. When you are exposed to the sun's harmful rays, melanin forms a cap over the nucleus of your skin cell to protect you from sun damage. Yes, a tan is really your skin telling you it's been sun-damaged. With chronically sun-exposed skin, the density of melanocytes increases, as does the production of pigment resulting in age spots and uneven pigmentation.

Melanocytes can also group together to form growths. A mole or nevus is a collection of normal-appearing melanocytes located in your epidermis or your dermis. A melanoma, on the other hand, is a collection of abnormal-appearing melanocytes, which grow in an uncontrolled fashion. Melanoma is the deadliest form of skin cancer, and like NMSC, is strongly linked to ultraviolet radiation from the sun as well as tanning beds.

The Dermis

The dermis is the middle layer of your skin. The dermis, like the epidermis, varies in thickness according to skin site, thinner on the face and thicker on the back. It's made mostly from collagen, elastin and hyaluronic acid which function to cushion the body from stress and strain and give your skin a youthful appearance. The leading role of your dermis is played by collagen. Collagen, a strong fibrous protein, serves as the major structural protein for the entire body. Collagen fibers are organized as parallel bands which are held together by elastin, acting like the bricks and mortar of your skin. Collagen is rich in the amino acids glycine, proline and lysine, as well as several other amino acids that are derived from protein sources in your diet. A diet lacking in protein-containing foods such as fish, eggs, meats, beans, nuts, and seeds, as well as vitamins and minerals including vitamin C, iron, zinc, and manganese interferes with the production of healthy collagen.

Collagen is most abundant in childhood which is why we all had those cheeks grandma loved to pinch. Gradually collagen production slows down in your thirties which is when you typically begin to sees signs of aging. Coupled with damage from sun exposure, environmental toxins, and nutritional deficiencies, the quality of your collagen may diminish, causing your skin to look saggy, leathery and wrinkled.

Elastin is what gives your skin its elasticity, allowing your skin to bounce back and maintain its youthful appearance. Hyaluronic acid is a sugar that binds water and retains moisture, which makes your face look supple and hydrated.

Taken all together, youthful skin has an abundance of collagen, elastin and hyaluronic acid. However, as these components decrease with age, the skin begins to appear thinner, saggier, drier and more wrinkled. This is why many popular skincare products contain these ingredients and dermal fillers, many of which are made of hyaluronic acid.

The dermis also contains fibroblasts that make collagen and elastin, sweat glands, sebaceous glands, hair follicles, blood vessels, lymphatic vessels and nerve bundles providing detoxification, protection, nourishment, and sensation to the epidermis. Your sebaceous glands secrete an oily substance called sebum, which lubricates and hydrates your skin. When overactive, your sebaceous glands can contribute to acne; when underactive, to dry, irritated skin.

The Subcutis

Beneath the dermis lies the subcutis, which is comprised of fat, connective tissue and blood vessels. Just like the epidermis and dermis, the subcutis varies in thickness according to skin site. The subcutis provides support and a source of energy, influences how we react to food and functions as an endocrine organ. The subcutis not only plays a role in hormone conversion, but the hormone leptin that regulates body weight is produced in your fat cells.

WHAT'S YOUR TYPE?

Yes, we all have a skin type. There is no good or bad, but knowing what type of skin you are in will empower you to know how to protect it best. Do you know your type?

In dermatology, we use a skin typing scale called the Fitzpatrick Skin Scale named after its creator, dermatologist Dr. Thomas Fitzpatrick. It is a numerical classification scheme which takes into account your hair, eye and skin color as well your interpretation of how your skin responds to the sun as a means to determine your skin cancer risk.

For example, if you are a fair-skinned individual with low levels of melanin in your epidermis, you tend to be more sun-sensitive with a susceptibility to burn rather than tan after ultraviolet light (UV) exposure. Not only are you less able to block UV radiation if you have fair skin, but UV exposure can cause harmful permanent changes to your DNA called *mutations*. What's more: the DNA repair mechanisms become defective. Taken together, these factors increase your risk of skin cancer.

So what's your type? Let's find out!

WHAT TYPE OF SKIN ARE YOU IN?

The Fitzpatrick Skin Scale is a skin classification system used to determine the skin's response to UV exposure using genetic factors and how the skin responds to UV radiation. Take the quiz to discover your type which can range from very fair [Type I] to very dark [Type VI]. Once complete, tally up your score and find your type. Then head to the website to collect your bonus skin type analysis and for some sun safety tips tailored to your skin type.

Source: Adapted from Skin Cancer Foundation

Part I: Genetic Predisposition
Your eye color is:

- Light blue, light gray or light green = 0 points
- Blue, gray or green = 1 points
- Hazel or light brown = 2 points
- Dark brown = 3 points
- Brownish black = 4 points

Your natural hair color is:

- Red or light blonde = 0 points
- Blonde = 1 points
- Dark blonde or light brown = 2 points
- Dark brown = 3 points
- Black = 4 points

Your natural skin color (before sun exposure) is:

- Ivory white = 0 points
- Fair or pale = 1 points

Fair to beige, with golden undertone = 2 points

Olive or light brown = 3 points

Dark brown or black = 4 points

How many freckles do you have on unexposed areas of your skin?

Many = 0 points

Several = 1 points

A few = 2 points

Very few = 3 points

None = 4 points

Total score for genetic disposition: _____

Part II: Reaction to Prolonged Sun Exposure

How does your skin respond to the sun?

Always burns, blisters and peels = 0 points

Often burns, blisters and peels = 1 points

Burns moderately = 2 points

Burns rarely, if at all = 3 points

Never burns = 4 points

Does your skin tan?

Never -- I always burn = 0 points

Seldom = 1 points

Sometimes = 2 points

Often = 3 points

Always = 4 points

How deeply do you tan?

Not at all or very little = 0 points

Lightly = 1 points

Moderately = 2 points

Deeply = 3 points

My skin is naturally dark = 4 points

How sensitive is your face to the sun?

Very sensitive = 0 points

Sensitive = 1 points

Normal = 2 points

Resistant = 3 points

Very resistant/Never had a problem = 4 points

Total score for reaction to prolonged sun exposure: _____

Add up your genetic disposition and sun exposure totals.

This is your Fitzpatrick Skin Type: _____

Results

Skin Type I (0-6 points): Mirror, mirror on the wall, you're the fairest of them all! Your skin always burns and never tans in the sun. Take extra precautions as you are extremely susceptible to skin damage.

Skin Type II (7-12 points): Not quite as fair as type I, your skin is still extremely vulnerable to the sun's harmful rays. Your skin almost always burns and rarely tans in the sun.

Skin Type III (13-18 points): You may see that bronzing eventually, but your skin is still very vulnerable to the sun's harmful rays. As a type III, your skin sometimes burns and sometimes tans in the sun.

Skin Type IV (19-24 points): Your skin tends to tan easily and is less likely to burn but you are still at risk and need to take care of the skin you're in.

Skin Type V (25-30 points): Sunburns may rarely be a concern as your skin tans easily, but you are still at risk for skin damage.

Skin Type VI (31+ points): Sunburns may not be in your vocabulary, as your skin never burns nor tans, but your skin is still vulnerable to the sun's harmful rays.

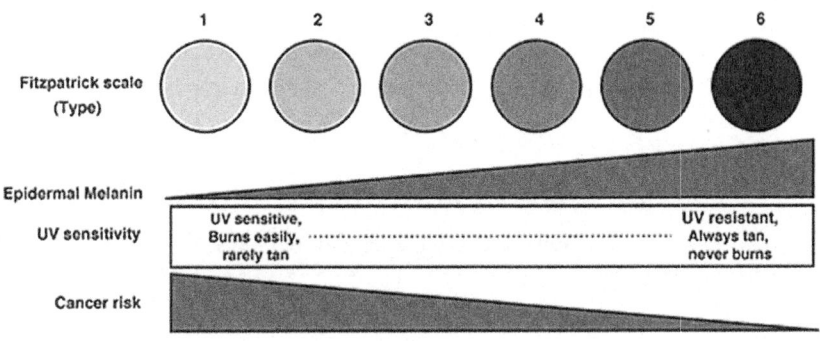

No matter what skin type you are, here's what is important to know: There are factors that influence your response to the sun and make you more sun-sensitive. These can include but are not limited to:

- autoimmune conditions (like lupus erythematosus and vitiligo)
- medications (such as certain antibiotics, blood pressure drugs, oral and topical retinoids)
- topical application of products containing ingredients, like citrus, or bergamot oil.

A word of warning! Be sure to check the labels of your medications and personal care products for warnings of increased sun sensitivity.

Keep in mind this skin type quiz is not intended to be a substitute for professional medical advice, diagnosis, or treatment. Always seek the advice of your physician or other qualified health provider with any questions you may have regarding a medical condition.

Swift Skin Action

Want more details on specific recommendations for your skin type?

Visit **www.drskinwhisperer.com**
to get the detailed analysis.

WHAT IMPACTS THE APPEARANCE OF THE SKIN YOU'RE IN?

Your skin is your armor. It is your first line of defense between you and the outside world, which means it is constantly getting pummeled by your environment and by your treatment of it. With time and exposure, you can develop chinks in your armor.

Aging occurs because of two different factors: intrinsic and extrinsic. You don't have much control over intrinsic factors, which are influenced by your genes, ethnicity and certain medical conditions. Although you may not be able to do much to change your intrinsic factors, there is great news! You can have a **huge impact** on your extrinsic factors which are major contributors to the aging process.

The most significant factor causing extrinsic aging is UV exposure. It is responsible for 90% of the visible signs of aging as well as significantly increasing your risk of melanoma skin cancer, and basal cell and squamous cell carcinomas, referred to as non-melanoma skin cancers. Of course, while you can't totally avoid going outside and exposing your skin to the elements, there are things you can do to minimize their impact. I'll go into more detail about UV exposure in Chapter 3.

The other major factors that cause extrinsic aging are:

- air pollution
- stress
- smoking
- diet
- lifestyle choices

With regards to stress, dietary and lifestyle choices, no worries, I've got you covered there too later in the book. Washing your

21

face twice daily, especially at night with a gentle cleanser to rinse away the daily grime and the air pollutants including polyaromatic hydrocarbons known to contribute to aging, pigmentation and acneiform eruptions will help minimize the effects As for smoking, the memo that it contributes to lung disease, cancer, skin aging and an overall abysmal state of health came out a long time ago. My hope is that you got that memo and either kicked cigarettes to the curb or never even picked them up.

HOW DO EXTRINSIC FACTORS IMPACT YOUR SKIN?

The combination and cumulative effect of the extrinsic factors that you're exposed to on a daily basis cause problems for your body and your skin in two major ways: through the formation of advanced glycation end products (AGEs) and free radicals. The formation of these two elements triggers a series of reactions causing inflammation in your body, damaging your cells and inhibiting their ability to function properly. The end result is DNA damage that can contribute to disease or worse… cancer.

WHAT ARE AGEs?

There is no denying that your body and skin need sugar (glucose) as fuel to function, but like with most things, there needs to be a **balance** for optimal performance.

All the food you eat gets converted into glucose, which is the simplest form of sugar that your body can use for energy. Foods containing more sugar as well as foods that are more readily converted into sugar like carbohydrates can flood your system with glucose. Foods with refined sugars like high fructose corn syrup, cane sugar, artificial sweeteners, and sugary products like soda, packaged cookies, cereals, and sauces can really increase the amount of sugar in your system. Any glucose that you don't need for energy right away gets stored in your liver and muscles as glycogen, a form of sugar that your body can use later when it needs more energy. When your liver and muscles have all of the glycogen they need, the leftover gets stored in your fat cells.

As you may know, the more sugar you eat, the more likely you are to increase your body fat. Maybe those bags of Halloween candy won't look as appetizing next year, eh? For most of us, in general, adding body fat is neither healthy nor desirable, yet the bigger issue with eating too much sugar is the impact it has on your insulin levels. When you eat food and your body converts it into glucose, your blood sugar rises and your body normally releases enough insulin to drive that extra sugar into your liver, muscles and fat cells for storage. When you consume a large amount of sugar, however, your body gets overwhelmed and chaos ensues. Instead of releasing a relatively small amount of insulin, your body floods your system with insulin in an attempt to drive your blood sugar down. The problem is that it can cause your blood sugar to become too low. Your body is then on a rollercoaster of high and low blood sugar spikes and labile insulin levels, which can lead to diabetes, obesity and inflammation.

Chronic inflammation is at the root of chronic disease system-wide and your skin is no exception. Inflammation can worsen rosacea, psoriasis, and eczema and may also weaken the collagen and elastin in your skin over time.

One of the other downsides of high blood sugar triggering insulin is that it in turn triggers insulin-like growth factor-1 (IGF-1). Both insulin and IGF-1 stimulate production of your androgen hormones, which turn your oil glands on, contributing to oily skin and worsening acne. Dairy, skim milk in particular, has been found to readily stimulate IGF-1, which is why I recommend a trial elimination of dairy when trying to get acne under control.

Okay, so we know sugar can make you gain weight and break out, but that's not all. One of the most significant impacts sugar has on the skin and on your body as a whole in regards to aging is through the process known as glycation. When high levels of sugar enter the circulation, they attach themselves to proteins and fats in your body, deforming them and causing them to malfunction. In your skin, glycation affects your collagen and elastin fibers. When sugar attaches to those, they form advanced glycation end products, also referred to as AGEs. AGEs cause your collagen and elastin to become stiff, inflexible, and prone to breakage. The result? Your skin becomes less elastic, wrinkled, saggy and more vulnerable to sun damage.

Although glycation is a normal process that occurs throughout the body and the skin, it is accelerated by a high-glycemic diet, cooking food at high temperatures (above 350 degrees) and excessive sun exposure. Glycation not only interferes with the function of collagen, but also stimulates the production of enzymes that break down collagen. This is a double whammy that increases the appearance of wrinkles and impairs wound healing. In Chapter 4, I'll talk more about the kinds of food to eat for younger and healthier looking skin.

The effects are more than just skin deep. While wrinkled skin is one of the visible signs of AGEs, most degenerative diseases are impacted on some level by disease-producing glycation reactions. These reactions can result in serious damage to your body, including heart disease, cataract formation, diabetes, cancer and even Alzheimer's disease. From your head to your feet, AGEs play a role in the aging process and their formation causes damage to your insides as well as your outsides. And sugar is the primary culprit.

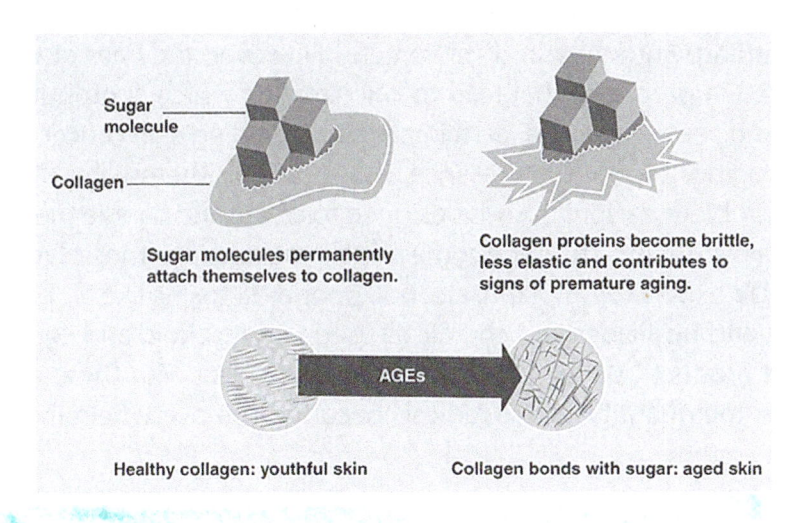

Sugar molecule

Collagen

Sugar molecules permanently attach themselves to collagen.

Collagen proteins become brittle, less elastic and contributes to signs of premature aging.

AGEs

Healthy collagen: youthful skin

Collagen bonds with sugar: aged skin

WHAT ARE FREE RADICALS?

Chemical reactions are happening outside and inside your body all the time, especially those that involve oxygen.

Let's look at the evidence. A slice of avocado, for example, soon turns brown if left in the open air. Rust can appear on a car that is exposed to the elements, due to the process of oxidation.

In your body, oxidation can be caused by AGEs and by molecules called **free radicals**. Free radicals are best described as unstable oxygen molecules that are missing at least one of their electrons. The thing is electrons like being paired up, so free radicals try to steal an electron from nearby cells in your body to make a pair. This causes oxidation of that cell resulting in cell and DNA damage or even cell death.

Your body produces free radicals all the time as a normal part of the making and functioning of your cells. Many of the processes involved in creating free radicals are beneficial, including digestion, breathing, immunity and movement. However, they are also involved in processes that lead to cell damage, which contribute to heart disease, cataracts, certain cancers including skin cancer, and skin aging. It is not the presence of free radicals themselves that is the problem, as your body is designed to create and handle them in certain amounts. The issue comes when you add in extrinsic factors like UV exposure, smoking, alcohol, poor diet, toxins like air pollution, and pesticides and chemicals used in household and agricultural products. When your body is trying to deal with these all at once, the quantity of free radicals becomes too overwhelming for your system.

The outcome is that your body enters a state of **oxidative stress**. It is unable to fight off the free radical damage on its own. Free radicals set off a chain of events in your body that begin to cause visible damage, including breakdown of your collagen and elastin. This makes your skin wrinkle, sag and appear thinner. And remember, as we age, collagen production is already slowing down, which accelerates if you combine that natural aging with extrinsic forces.

Although you cannot avoid free radicals, the damage they cause can be greatly reduced by a diet and skincare routine rich in **antioxidants**. Antioxidants are the antidote to free radicals. Vitamins A, C, E, anthocyanins, beta-carotene, lycopene, zinc, selenium and resveratrol are just a few of the antioxidants that serve to protect your skin and your body by donating one of their electrons to the free radical so it can no longer cause damage. Your body produces a natural reserve of antioxidants, including glutathione and superoxide dismutase, but your supply can become quickly depleted when faced with a barrage of extrinsic factors.

The good news is that by eating foods, incorporating select supplements and using skincare products rich in antioxidants, you can help replenish your reserve. I'll talk a lot more about how to best nourish your body and skin in Chapter 4.

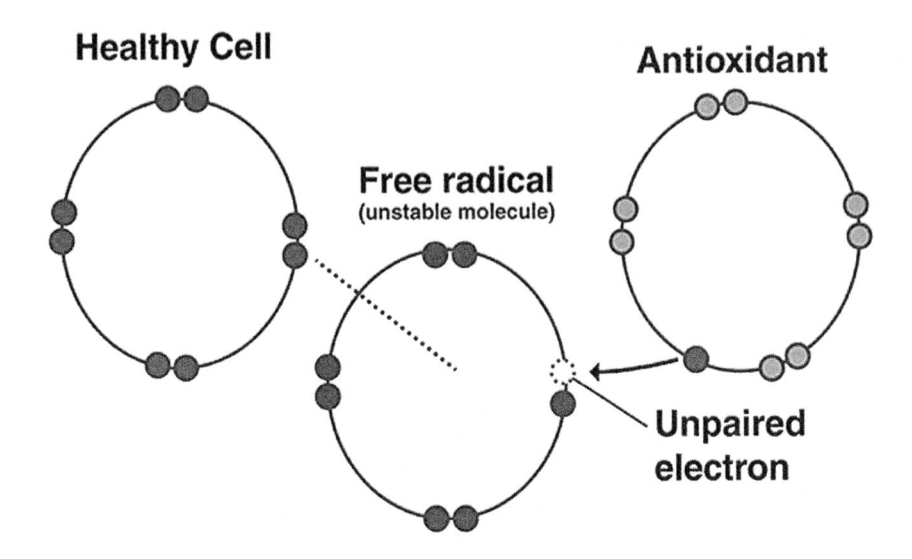

Healthy Cell — **Free radical** (unstable molecule) — **Antioxidant** — **Unpaired electron**

PUTTING IT ALL TOGETHER: HOW TO EXAMINE THE SKIN YOU'RE IN

As a dermatologist, what I love about the human body is that your hair, nails and skin can provide a **wealth of information** as to the status of your health, both present and past. By getting to know the skin you're in, you can be your own detective to gather clues to optimize your wellness, slow down the clock and feel like the rockstar you are!

Below are my recommendations for getting ready to party in your birthday suit! The only way to examine your skin is to see it. All of it. Don't be modest. Get naked and have fun with it. You know your body better than anyone else, and you're going to be the one to notice when things are growing, changing, or behaving differently from how they have before.

When you take notice, you can take action.

Here's what to do:

- Make a date with yourself. Pick one day a month that you commit to checking your skin and put it in your calendar. I recommend the date of your birthday as a good reminder to check your birthday suit!

- Get naked. Keep it simple and examine yourself either before or after your shower. You're already naked, so make the most of it. Check your birthday suit and look for any uninvited guests!

- Top to bottom: Start at the top of your head and work your way down to your toes. Look in all your nooks and crannies: your mouth, lips, ears, armpits, belly button, nails, between your fingers and toes, the tops and bottoms of your feet.

- Check out your intimate bits — front and back. I mean really check them. Grab a hand mirror so you can see the skin externally and internally.

Skin is skin so check all of it. For places you can't easily see, don't be shy… recruit help. Get your hairstylist to look on your scalp. Get your ophthalmologist to look in your eyes. Get your dentist to look in your mouth. Ask your OB/GYN to check you where the sun doesn't shine.

Skin cancers and other lesions can occur in covered areas, so it behooves you to check every inch of yourself. Take pictures so you can compare what you are seeing from month to month.

SO WHAT ARE YOU LOOKING FOR?

Given my personal and professional experience, I want to be absolutely certain you know how to check your skin is healthy, especially for signs of skin cancer. There are two methods for doing this. While I recommend using both, the second one may be easier. You are going to examine every inch of yourself with either method so you won't miss a thing.

The first method is more applicable for checking your skin to differentiate between moles/nevi and melanoma skin cancer. In this method, you are going to use the ABCDE principles for checking your "spots."

A is for *asymmetry*. With regards to a spot, you want to be able to visually cut it down the middle and have it look the same on both sides.

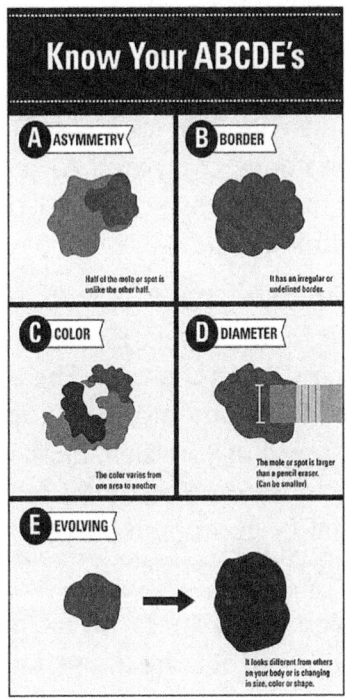

Know Your ABCDE's

A ASYMMETRY
Half of the mole or spot is unlike the other half.

B BORDER
It has an irregular or undefined border.

C COLOR
The color varies from one area to another

D DIAMETER
The mole or spot is larger than a pencil eraser. (Can be smaller)

E EVOLVING
It looks different from others on your body or is changing in size, color or shape.

B is for **border**. A spot should have a uniform, sharply demarcated border. You don't want to see irregular, scalloped or poorly defined margins.

C is for **color**. There should be uniformity of color throughout the spot. Typically moles are shades of brown. Though there are blue nevi and flesh-colored nevi as well. What you don't want to see is a mole that has multiple colors within it. It doesn't always mean that something is wrong, but it does mean you should get that particular spot checked by your dermatologist.

D is for **diameter**. The classic teaching is you want a spot to be less than the size of a pencil eraser which is approximately 5mm. In my opinion, this feature is not always as useful, because I have seen melanomas that have been much smaller than this. That said, a new or changing spot that is much larger than this is one you should get checked out.

E is for **evolving**. This is by far the most important principle and I encourage you to put your emphasis on checking this aspect of your skin. You are looking for any spot that has changed in size, color, and appearance compared to your last exam. If you suspect any of your spots to have changed, please seek the assistance of your dermatologist.

The second method is what is known as the "ugly duckling" sign. Put simply, the "ugly duckling" is any spot or finding that stands out from the rest of your crowd. The utility of this method is that it can be applied to pigmented and non-pigmented lesions, as well as the appearance of your hair, nails, and any part of your skin. You are looking for something that is out of place either from your baseline normal or compared to your last exam. In other words, you are looking for patterns.

As regards to pigmented spots, for example, you may find a pattern that you have small or large moles, or they are light brown or dark brown in color. When you find a spot that doesn't fit your pattern, that is your "ugly duckling." This method is also very helpful to check for the non-melanoma skin cancers (NMSC), basal cell carcinomas (BCC) and squamous cell carcinomas (SCC), as well as the precursor to skin cancer called actinic keratosis.

BCC comes in several different forms and can present as a pearly bump, a reddish scaly patch or a sore that isn't healing.

SCC can present in a very similar way, as a scaly red patch or non-healing sore, but instead of a pearly bump, SCC could look like a heaped up mound of tissue resembling a volcano about to erupt. The latter type of SCC often presents on the arms and legs.

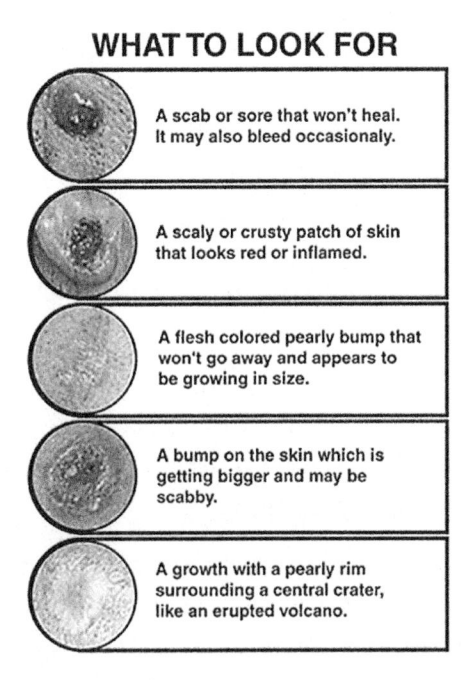

WHAT TO LOOK FOR

- A scab or sore that won't heal. It may also bleed occasionaly.
- A scaly or crusty patch of skin that looks red or inflamed.
- A flesh colored pearly bump that won't go away and appears to be growing in size.
- A bump on the skin which is getting bigger and may be scabby.
- A growth with a pearly rim surrounding a central crater, like an erupted volcano.

Actinic keratoses are precursors to SCC and can often be felt more than they can be seen. They feel like gritty sandpaper and may have a pink to reddish hue. They occur on chronically sun-exposed body parts, including the head, neck, hands, arms, and legs. Compared to your normal skin, any of these findings would stand out from your crowd. They would be considered "ugly ducklings" and should be checked by your dermatologist.

Because skin cell turnover time is short, occurring every few weeks, the appearance of your skin is an excellent mirror of your overall nutritional status.

Nutritional deficiencies including vitamin, mineral and protein deficiencies can lead to brittle nails, hair loss, flare-ups of inflammatory skin issues, poor wound healing, as well as cancer formation. While it may be a single nutrient deficiency, it is not uncommon for there to be multiple and what you see on your skin can be a reflection of this. Although it is not always possible to pinpoint the full spectrum of deficiencies on visual inspection alone, by taking notice of the quality and condition of your hair, skin and nails you may find your "ugly duckling" and that can provide clues to something happening deeper in your body. These clues enable you to **take control** of your health and seek help from your physician.

Now that you understand a little bit more about your skin, I want you to get familiar with it. Your skin is not trying to sabotage you. It truly is trying to protect you and alert you to what is happening on the inside of your body.

When your skin is dry or a little irritated, that's your skin whispering to you. When you have thinning hair or you notice consistent irritation and inflammation, your body is talking a little bit louder. If you have a growing and changing pigmented lesion or a sore that's not healing, that's your skin trying to shout at you. It's important that you **pay attention**, because a skin cancer diagnosis is no joke.

Remember, you are not in this alone! I recommend you get a full body skin exam performed by a board-certified dermatologist at least once a year. During the rest of the year, put a self-check date on your calendar every month.

What to do if you find an uninvited guest on your birthday suit? When in doubt, get it checked out by a board certified dermatologist. Visit the American Academy of Dermatology website to find a dermatologist near you. Better yet, ask your friends and family for a recommendation of someone they know and trust.

Swift Skin Action
Get these graphics as printables and keep the information on hand.

www.drskinwhisperer.com

Chapter 3:
WHY SPF ISN'T YOUR ONLY BFF

"When you put all your eggs in one basket, you've got a problem."

Ander Crenshaw

As a kid, SPF and sunscreen weren't a regular part of my vocabulary. Actually, back then it was called suntan oil and my sister and I would have contests to see how low we could go with the SPF! The winner would go without sunscreen at all... Being a fair-skinned brunette, the suntan oil on my skin just amplified my tendency to burn. Although I would tan eventually, the pain of the sunburn, followed by the accumulation of freckles and moles made me a loser every time.

If I had known then what I know now, skin cancer wouldn't be part of my personal vocabulary; it would have been strictly professional. But here's the thing you need to know. The most prevalent cancer is the **most preventable** and the most ignored. Skin cancer is the most widespread cancer in the United States and around the world.

SKIN CANCER FACTS

- Each year in the U.S., there are more new cases of skin cancer than the incidence of breast, prostate, lung and colon cancers combined.
- Over 5 million cases are diagnosed in more than 3 million people every year.
- One in five Americans will develop skin cancer during their lifetime.
- There are three main types of skin cancers — basal cell carcinoma (BCC), squamous cell carcinoma (SCC) and melanoma — named after the skin cell type from which they are derived.
- BCC and SCC are the two major forms of non-melanoma skin cancer. BCC is the most common and SCC is second. 40-50% of Americans over the age of 65 will have either one at least once.
- Most BCCs and SCCs occur in chronically sun-exposed areas including the face, neck and arms. Melanomas tend to present on intermittently sun-exposed areas such as the back and calves.
- Melanoma, though only comprising 5% of all skin cancers, is the most deadly form.
- 90% of NMSCs and 86% of melanomas are associated with sun exposure. Tanning increases your rate of skin cancer by 75%, which is why tanning beds are a carcinogen just like cigarettes.
- About 90% of the visible changes commonly attributed to aging are caused by sun exposure.
- It costs over $8 billion USD annually to treat and those numbers continue to rise.

Bottom line: This is not only a **public health issue**; it is a significant financial **drain on our society**. But there is something we can do about. There is something *you* can do about it.

I want to share the facts with you, dispel the myths and make sure you know how to prepare and protect yourself while having fun in the sun. Yes! That's right. You don't have to be a hermit! Getting outside in nature is so important on many levels. Life is meant to be enjoyed. Adventures are meant to be had. And that includes soaking up the energy and abundant joy that sunlight provides us. I'm here to help you empower yourself with the knowledge and skills you need to reduce the risk factors while increasing protective factors associated with skin cancer and aging so you can look younger, radiate your beauty and live life outdoors to the fullest. Protecting your skin not only keeps you looking younger, but it can save your life.

When it comes to perspective about ultraviolet radiation (UVR) exposure, Greek mythology provides a great example. Apollo was the Olympian god of music, healing, sun and light as well as the protector of the young — but Apollo could also bring sickness as powerfully as he could bring cure. In our daily lives, our exposure to the sun has a similar duality. Without the sun, life on Earth could not exist. Sunlight is essential to the survival of our plants and wildlife. It plays a significant role in our immune function, our skin's ability to generate vitamin D. And it produces endorphins, those feel-good hormones that makes us so attracted to its warmth and glow. That said, extensive and chronic UVR exposure causes mayhem for the skin. It induces local as well as systemic suppression of your immune system, weakening your ability to deal with the solar assault, while simultaneously generating AGEs and free radicals, which are unstable oxygen molecules disrupting cell function, producing inflammation and damaging your skin's DNA. By suppressing your immune system, UVR also alters responses to infectious agents and your body's ability to protect itself. UVR packs a potent punch because it not only damages your skin's DNA directly and indirectly with ultraviolet B (UVB) and ultraviolet A (UVA) rays respectively, it also interferes with your skin's DNA repair mechanisms. Talk about a double whammy!

Your body is equipped with a pretty sophisticated defense system, which includes antioxidants to fend off the generation of free radicals and reactive oxygen species. However, your body's reserve of these substances is not unlimited, and at some point, your system gets depleted.

What does this all mean?

It means that if there is an imbalance between UV-induced DNA damage and your body's ability to repair it, mutations can occur in your genes, which lead to skin cancer.

What is the deal with sunlight?

Sunlight consists of a spectrum of electromagnetic rays with different wavelengths, energy values and depth of penetration into the skin: visible light (VL), infrared light (IR) and ultraviolet light (UVR). VL accounts for 50% of the sunlight spectrum and, as the name suggests, can be detected by the human eye. With a wavelength range of 400 to 760 nanometers (nm), VL penetrates deep into the dermis and subcutis. While visible light is used clinically for the treatment of a variety of skin diseases and esthetic conditions in the form of lasers, intense pulsed light and photodynamic therapy, recent studies have shown it can damage the skin as well. VL causes indirect DNA damage through the generation of reactive oxygen species, and contributes to photodermatoses which are a group of skin disorders triggered by sunlight exposure. IR, invisible to the eye, represents 45% of the solar spectrum and is divided into three groups according to wavelength; IRA (740–1400 nm), IRB (1400–3000 nm) and IRC (3000 nm–1 mm). While IRB and IRC do not penetrate the skin deeply, IRA which represents the majority of the IR spectrum penetrates deep into the dermis and subcutis like VL. Although they don't pack as powerful a punch as UVR, recent studies have shown that VL and IR decrease collagen production, induce breakdown of dermal tissue, compromise skin barrier function and contribute to increased skin pigmentation.

UVR, also invisible to the human eye, accounts for the remaining 5% of the solar spectrum that is comprised of UVA (315-400 nm), UVB (280-315 nm) and UVC (100-280 nm) rays. Fortunately, UVC rays, the most damaging ones, are largely absorbed by the ozone layer and do not typically reach Earth's surface, so it's the UVA and UVB rays that cause the majority of effects on the skin, both short and long term. UVB rays, shorter in wavelength, penetrate the epidermis and upper dermis. Their intensity varies with time of day (strongest between 10am and 4pm), season, latitude, longitude, altitude and reflection off surfaces including water, snow and pavement. In fact, for every 1,000 feet of elevation, the intensity of UVB increases by 10%. Have you ever noticed people in the ski lodge whose faces are burned to a crisp? It's because of the combination of more potent UVB rays plus their reflection off the snow. It's like getting blasted by the sun twice. UVB rays are also blocked by window glass.

Longer in wavelength, UVA rays penetrate deeply into the dermis, can penetrate window glass and have consistent intensity throughout the year. As a driver, have you noticed that your face and arm on one side have more wrinkles and mottled pigmentation than the other side? Those UVA rays penetrating your driver's side window are the culprit.

The short-term effects of UVR on the skin include sunburn and tanning. UVB rays are primarily responsible for causing sunburns. They are often referred to as the "burning rays." Both UVB and UVA rays contribute to tanning.

One of the most important long-term associations of UV damage, certainly, is the risk of skin cancer. UVR is considered a **complete carcinogen**, which means it is capable of initiating, promoting and advancing the progression of cancer cells by directly and indirectly damaging DNA. The most important defense mechanisms the skin has to protect itself are melanin production and active repair mechanisms. In fact, a tan is your body's attempt to shield your cells' DNA from the damaging effects of the sun. Together, UVA and UVB rays generate free radicals, cellular and DNA damage as well as suppression of the immune system resulting in sunburn, pigment changes, risk of skin cancer development and eye damage (including cataracts and ocular melanoma).

Another important long-term effect of UVR is its contribution to premature skin aging, also known as photoaging. With 90% of the visible signs of aging including skin sagging, wrinkles, dilated blood vessels, mottled pigmentation and a leathery appearance attributed to sun exposure, protecting yourself from the sun every day is your ticket to youthful skin.

When UV rays hit the skin, it sets off a sequence. One, your epidermis scrambles to shield cellular DNA with melanin resulting in mottled pigmentation. When the skin's ability to manufacture its own protection is overwhelmed, DNA damage occurs. Two, because UVA rays can penetrate deep into the dermis, they damage the collagen and elastin through production of AGEs. The AGEs bind to the proteins of collagen and elastin rendering these fibers stiff and dysfunctional. This damage also leads to increased production of abnormal elastic fibers. As the process repeats with daily UVA exposure, the damaged fibers create wrinkles, and the depleted collagen manifests as leathery skin.

What can you do about it?

1. Minimize your exposure when the UVB rays' intensity is the greatest between 10am and 4pm.
2. Seek shade. If your shadow is shorter than you, the sun's intensity is strong and you should take cover.
3. Accessorize! Wear a hat with at least a 4-inch brim and wear sunglasses that offer protection from both UVA and UVB rays.
4. Wear protective clothing. The Skin Cancer Foundation ranks clothing as **the single most effective** form of sun protection. By limiting the amount of skin exposure by covering yourself with clothes, you minimize your risk.
5. Wear sunscreen. Topically applied sunscreens offer protection by reflecting or absorbing UVR at the skin surface.

Most dermatologists will tell you that sunscreen is your first line of defense. Here's where I take a stand. While I think SPF should be in your inner circle, it should not be your only BFF when it comes to protecting your skin. It is true that sunscreens have been thoroughly researched in the scientific literature and have been shown to prevent skin cancers, sunburns and photoaging. They're an important part of a comprehensive sun protection strategy, no doubt. In fact, I always tell my patients that using sunscreen should be like brushing your teeth: a *part* of your non-negotiable daily routine. Why? Because the benefits can only be realized if people actually use them as intended on a consistent basis. Even on overcast days, up to 80% of UV rays penetrate the clouds. With less than half of the

The Skin Whisperer

US population regularly applying sunscreen, there are plenty of people not experiencing the benefits. That said, just like brushing alone doesn't guarantee optimal oral health, the use of sunscreen alone cannot prevent development of skin cancer.

How do you choose the best protective clothing?

Similar to creating fine wine, clothing that provides effective sun protection requires multiple factors to be present. These factors include color, weight, weave, whether the clothing is wet or dry, and if it has been washed. The color of the clothing determines how easily sunlight can get through it. Darker clothing is better at blocking the sun's rays. Next, choose clothing with a greater weight so that there is more material to absorb more UV rays. The weave is also important. The tighter the knit or weave, the smaller the spaces between fibers and the less UVR getting through. Fabric composed of synthetic fibers such as polyester, Lycra and nylon offer greater protection than cotton. That said, when it comes to cotton, washing and putting it through a dryer will tighten the weave and make the clothing more protective. Taken together, we can consider these factors and use them to measure the sun protection that clothing products provide, referred to as UPF (ultraviolet protection factor). UPF ratings indicate how much UV can penetrate the fabric. For instance, a shirt with a UPF 50 allows just one-fiftieth (1/50) of the sun's UV radiation to reach your skin, which is considered excellent protection. Let's put it in perspective. Your basic cotton t-shirt provides a UPF ~5. Keep in mind that this can decrease; both tension on fabric (stretch from tight-fitting clothing) and moisture can decrease the UPF rating of any fabric.

So what do you do when heading outdoors and want to play it safe? Keep it simple: cover up as much of your exposed skin with loose-fitting, lightweight, tightly woven fabrics in darker colors. If you can find UPF-rated clothing that fits your style choose UPF 30-50 to provide you with the best protection.

Why you should put sunscreen on your daily to-do list

1. Sunscreen has been proven to decrease the development of skin cancer.

2. More than five sunburns in a person's lifetime, regardless of timing, doubles the risk of developing melanoma.

3. Sunscreen helps to prevent skin discolorations, dilated blood vessels and blotchiness.

4. There are numerous medications that can make the skin more susceptible to the harmful effects of the sun and using sunscreen can minimize that risk. Anti-inflammatory, cardiovascular and acne medications are among the categories well-known to increase skin's vulnerability to a burn. For example, acne medications including oral doxycycline and minocycline, oral and topical vitamin A derivatives including isotretinoin (Accutane) and tretinoin (Retin-A), as well as benzoyl peroxide, may make certain skin types (such as Fitzpatrick Skin Types I through III) burn more easily through photosensitization and irritation, respectively.

5. Certain medical conditions can be triggered or exacerbated by direct and prolonged sun exposure including sun allergies like polymorphous light eruption and autoimmune conditions like lupus erythematosus. Sunscreen offers additional protection. For patients lacking protective melanin pigment, including those with vitiligo and albinism, a sunburn is absolutely inevitable without appropriate protection. Studies have also demonstrated benefits for organ transplant recipients regularly using broad-spectrum sunscreens to prevent the development of skin cancer, both its precursors and invasive forms.

6. Use of sunscreen slows down the development of sagging, wrinkling and prematurely aging skin.

Why sunscreen should not be all you use to protect yourself

1. Less than half of Americans reported that they regularly use sunscreen on both their face and other exposed skin when outside in the sun for more than an hour according to Centers for Disease Control and Prevention in 2013.

2. 68% of people don't know that SPF 30 sunscreen does not provide twice as much protection as an SPF 15 sunscreen according to a 2016 survey conducted by the American Academy of Dermatology (AAD).

3. 55% of people don't understand that a higher-SPF sunscreen does not protect you from the sun for longer than a lower-SPF sunscreen.

4. The Food and Drug Administration (FDA) has not approved any new sunscreen filters for formulations in over 10 years. As a consequence, there is concern that US sunscreen may not offer broad-spectrum UV protection comparable to those in other parts of the world. Moreover, ultraviolet filters in the majority of commercially available sunscreen do not protect against visible and infrared radiation which also damage skin and contribute to premature aging.

5. The majority of sunscreen users do not apply enough sunscreen to get the full SPF protection listed on label. Most people use only 25% to 50% of the recommended amount.

6. Most people are not reapplying sunscreen to get continued protection while they are outside in the sun longer than two hours.

There is no denying that sunscreen is an asset in your sun protective arsenal. I'm going to confront the controversies and share with you what you need to know about them. And yet, it's also important to understand that they aren't a magic potion that can provide all the protection you need, which is why I am a firm believer that you need to use them, but they should never be your first or only line of defense in the sun.

USING SUNSCREEN: THE BASICS

There are several key elements that can help with choosing the right sunscreen:

Ingredients

No matter which sunscreen you choose, make certain it is labeled as broad-spectrum protection, which means it can protect against both UVA and UVB radiation.

Physical vs. chemical

What is the difference between physical sunscreens and chemical sunscreens?

Physical sunscreens contain active mineral ingredients, such as titanium dioxide or zinc oxide, which work by sitting on top of the skin to deflect, scatter and block UV rays from reaching the skin surface. Zinc oxide in particular effectively protects against both UVA and UVB rays providing broad-spectrum coverage. These filters also remain more stable when exposed to UV rays, unlike many of the chemical UV filters that degrade in the sun.

They are active immediately upon application to the skin

and are the least likely to cause a reaction, making them a good choice for young children and those with sensitive skin. Although some formulations can leave a white cast on the skin, many are available without leaving traces of white pigment or causing irritation.

Chemical sunscreens use active ingredients such as avobenzone, oxybenzone, octinoxate and octisalate, which absorb UV radiation and create a chemical reaction by changing UV rays into heat which is then released from the skin. If you've ever noticed your skin feel warmer after applying sunscreen, this is why. Unlike physical filters, chemical filters require at least 20 minutes after application to become active and have a greater tendency to cause skin irritation and allergic contact dermatitis. Most chemical UV filters can only offer protection for UVA or UVB, but typically not both, which is why you will find sunscreens that contain both physical and chemical ingredients to provide broad-spectrum protection.

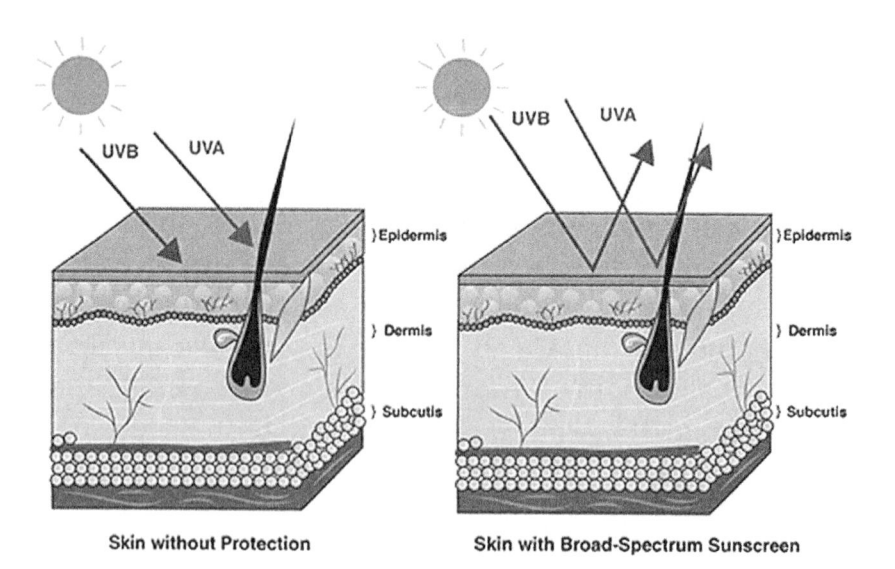

Skin without Protection

Skin with Broad-Spectrum Sunscreen

SPF

SPF stands for **sun protection factor** and is the standard measurement of a sunscreen's ability to protect you in the sun. While SPF ratings are important, SPF only refers to the protection against sunburns that are caused by UVB rays (and a small fraction of UVA).

How much UVB protection are you getting? SPF 15 blocks 93% of UVB rays; SPF 30 blocks 97%; SPF 50 blocks 98% and SPF 100 blocks 99%. As you can see there is no SPF that can offer 100% protection from UVB rays.

Using a higher SPF does not afford you that much more protection which is why the American Academy of Dermatology recommends using sunscreen with a minimum of SPF 30. That said, the actual SPF you get when applying sunscreen is determined by how much and how often you apply.

How much should you apply?

Sunscreen should be applied daily to areas not covered by clothing including on cloudy or overcast days. Up to 80% of those rays are still getting through those clouds. The recommended amount of sunscreen for your entire body is a minimum of 1 ounce (2 tablespoons) or the equivalent of a shot glass full of sunscreen. You may need more if you are very tall or have more skin exposed. For the face alone, approximately one third of a teaspoon should be used, with more needed to ensure coverage of your ears, neck and scalp. To cover them all, a safe estimate is one teaspoon. Studies have revealed that for any given SPF, most people apply between 25% and 50% of the recommended amount. The problem with this is users may have a false sense of security regarding the amount of protection they are actually getting, which may even encourage them to expose themselves to the sun's damaging rays for longer. Don't let this happen to you. Grab a shot glass and measure it out if you need to. There is no such thing as using too much, so apply liberally.

How often should you apply?

As most people don't apply the recommended dose the first time, it's a good idea to apply a second coat within 20 minutes to optimize your protection. The official recommendation is to reapply sunscreen every two hours due to degradation of the filters by the sun, as well as it wearing off from sweating, swimming and friction from clothing or towels. So if you have a 4-ounce bottle of sunscreen and you are at the beach a full day of eight hours, that bottle should be empty by the time you head home.

Water resistance

Not all sunscreens are tested for water resistance, which means when you are swimming or sweating, your sunscreen may be wearing off more quickly. Be sure to look on the bottle for the "water resistant" or "very water resistant" labels and note the time listed, which may range from 40 to 80 minutes. Always re-apply your sunscreen as soon as you get out of the pool or ocean, because the testing for these sunscreens is not done in chlorinated or salt water, and this may impact the sunscreen's usefulness.

There is one very important thing to keep in mind regarding labels that I want to bring to your attention. The FDA requires sunscreen manufacturers to test their own products, but the agency does not perform its own independent testing to verify the manufacturer's claims. This is why I am a big fan of the studies performed on sunscreens by Consumer Reports, which compile the results of extensive testing to verify that products work as they are advertised. These reports come out each Spring. For peace of mind and the safety of your skin, it's a good idea to check it out.

What form of sunscreen is best? What about sprays?

Here's the bottom line: the best form of sunscreen is the one you will use. Choose a sunscreen that feels good on your skin, does not cause irritation and that you will use consistently. That said, go for lotions and creams over sprays. The issue with sprays is that most of the spray winds up in the air, not on your skin, and the sunscreen won't be evenly distributed on your skin. It still requires that you make an effort to rub in the sunscreen thoroughly and cover your skin surface completely.

An additional issue relates to sprays and concern about inhalation of zinc oxide and titanium dioxide nanoparticles. The Environmental Working Group advises against using any spray or loose powder sunscreens that contain these ingredients to avoid the potential toxicity from inhalation. That said, there are many products on the market providing broad-spectrum coverage that do not contain nanoparticles so this does not have to be a concern.

THE MYTHS AND CONTROVERSIES

Does sunscreen cause skin cancer?

As the most prevalent cancer in the United States with ever-increasing rates coupled with the surge of sunscreens on the market, one may come to the conclusion that sunscreen use and cancer are linked, but it's not true. Studies have shown that sunscreen has not only reduced the number of moles accumulated from sun exposure, one of the risk factors for melanoma, but it has also reduced the risk of both melanoma and non-melanoma skin cancers themselves. Most skin cancers are preventable. Sunscreen should be a component of a comprehensive sun protection strategy.

So what gives? Here's the thing. Wearing sunscreen with SPF blocks the UVB rays that are the major contributor to sunburn. As the time to burn may be delayed by wearing sunscreen, this can provide users with a false sense of security of their level of protection. Even if the onset of a sunburn is delayed, UVB and UVA rays are still penetrating the skin and generating reactive oxygen species, free radicals with the potential for cellular and DNA damage. As noted above, the vast majority of users do not use the recommended amount of sunscreen to realize the full potential of their SPF; nor do they re-apply it often enough to continue to experience the benefit. Couple these factors with a cocktail or two poolside, which may divert attention away from keeping track of time outdoors (not to mention the alcohol's contribution to oxidative stress), and it's a recipe for sun damage and elevated cancer risk.

So you see, it's not the use of sunscreen itself, but how it's being used (or not) that contributes so highly to the rise of skin cancer. As skin-revealing clothing styles and tropical holidays have become the norm in our society, the amount of acute and intermittent sun exposure an individual gets over the course of their lifetime has increased exponentially compared to our ancestors whose clothing had greater coverage and who stayed closer to home. This is why BCC is the most common of the skin cancers, being most closely associated with **acute and intermittent sun exposure**.

Are sunscreens dangerous because of the nanoparticles?

In 1999, the FDA approved sunscreen to be formulated with nanoparticles. Nanoparticles are tiny particles that are less than 100 nanometers in diameter. Creating sunscreen with these minute particles allows for sunscreen ingredients like zinc oxide and titanium dioxide to be blended more easily and appear transparent rather than the traditional thick white paste.

To be honest, not as much is known about the long-term safety of using nanoparticle sunscreens, so it is understandable that consumers have concern about their use. Based on studies, zinc oxide nanoparticles in sunscreen do not penetrate the epidermis of healthy skin and are not thought to pose any danger. The role of titanium dioxide nanoparticles is unclear, as pilot studies show that they may penetrate to the dermis. For now, both zinc oxide and titanium dioxide are approved for use in the formulation of sunscreens, though further research needs to be done.

Non-nanoparticle-containing sunscreens with zinc oxide and titanium dioxide are readily available on the market. These are what I recommend you use. Make sure to read your labels as these products will be clearly marked "no nanoparticles" or "non-nano" on their packaging.

Do sunscreens cause endocrine disruption?

Several of the chemical filters used in sunscreens, including homosalate, octinoxate and oxybenzone have been detected in urine and breast milk, and found to have endocrine-disrupting effects on estrogen, progesterone, androgen, and thyroid hormone receptors. Oxybenzone was shown to mimic estrogen and be associated with endometriosis in women, as well as having high rates of allergic reactions.

Although the American Academy of Dermatology's position is that these sunscreens are safe, as there are no published studies showing sunscreen to be toxic to humans or hazardous to human health, current studies in the literature provide conflicting data. As chemical UV filters have a tendency to cause skin irritation and allergic reactions, out of personal preference and based on recent studies, I recommend exclusive use of physical UV filters with zinc oxide.

For more detailed information about most sunscreens on the market, go to www.ewg.org/skindeep

Does sunscreen cause vitamin D deficiency?

Vitamin D is vital to our health. Almost every cell in our body has a vitamin D receptor which, when bound to vitamin D, influences the expression of more than 1000 genes. Vitamin D is a hormone responsible for promoting strong bones, regulating immune function, cell growth, neuromuscular function, and maintaining calcium and phosphate levels in the blood. Healthy levels of vitamin D support digestive wellness and mood stability. That means less depression and a greater sense of wellbeing. Healthy levels of vitamin D have also been associated with decreasing risk of heart disease, diabetes, autoimmune disease and cancer. With regards to skin health, there are studies showing that vitamin D protects against the damaging effects of free radicals and reduces inflammation. A recent study in the Journal of Investigative Dermatology showed that oral supplementation of vitamin D can quickly reduce inflammation caused by a sunburn. There are even some studies suggesting higher levels of vitamin D may be protective against melanoma, and others finding benefits of supplementation for skin cancer prevention as well as companion therapy for managing melanoma.

What's more: the literature supports the notion that maintaining a vitamin D serum concentration within normal levels is warranted in a spectrum of skin conditions including atopic dermatitis, psoriasis, vitiligo, polymorphous light eruption, alopecia areata, systemic lupus erythematosus. Vitamin D is created when the ultraviolet rays of the sun act upon a form of cholesterol in the skin called 7-dehydrocholesterol (7-DHC). The UVB rays from the sun convert 7-DHC into the inactive precursor vitamin D3. From there, vitamin D3 travels through the bloodstream to the liver and then the kidneys to generate 1,25 dihydroxyvitamin D(calcitriol), the biologically active form of vitamin D. As sunscreen with higher SPF blocks UVB rays, concern has been raised that sunscreen use could potentially inhibit vitamin D production and be the culprit of vitamin D deficiency.

Here's the thing. Sunscreen, even at the highest SPF available, does not block 100% of UVB rays, and our skin is always getting some degree of sun exposure. More importantly, 50% of Americans do not consistently use sunscreen and those who do typically only apply 25 to 50% of the recommended amount, which means that a significant amount of UVB exposure is still penetrating the epidermis of most people using sunscreen.

Numerous studies have shown that sunscreen does not decrease vitamin D production enough to be a significant cause of deficiency. In fact, an Australian study showed that there was no difference in vitamin D levels between adults randomly assigned to use sunscreen in summertime and those given a placebo with no UVB-blocking ability.

The most significant determinants of vitamin D deficiency are related to your age, weight, skin color, where you live, genetics, diet and lifestyle factors.

Melanin competes with 7-DHC for the absorption of UV light acting as a natural sunscreen, which reduces the effectiveness of vitamin D production in skin. This means that individuals with dark-colored skin require more time (up to ten times as long) to synthesize the same amount of previtamin D3 in skin as those with people with fair skin. Aging impacts vitamin D synthesis since older adults have lower skin concentrations of 7-DHC, compared to younger individuals. Because cholesterol acts as a precursor to vitamin D creation, your body needs cholesterol to maintain healthy vitamin D levels. Eating a low cholesterol diet, whether it's by avoiding egg yolks or opting for "fat-free" foods, may result in not having enough cholesterol to produce sufficient levels of vitamin D. Couple that with the reality that it's challenging to get the amount of vitamin D you need through foods alone, even if you aren't on a low cholesterol diet.

Based on latitude and longitude, a significant proportion of the United States does not get sufficient UVB exposure most of the year to stimulate production of vitamin D. For example, those residing in temperate latitudes, around 40 degrees north or 40 degrees south (like Boston which is 42 degrees north), have inadequate UVB radiation available for vitamin D synthesis from November to early March. By moving just ten degrees farther north (like Edmonton, Canada) or south, the "vitamin D void" extends from October to April. Combine this with indoor occupations, sedentary indoor pastimes like scrolling social media, playing video games and watching TV, the vast majority of people are vitamin D deficient regardless of whether they use sunscreen or not.

To illustrate this point, studies show that indoor workers have a higher incidence of melanoma than outdoors workers. Let's look at why this might be. Window glass blocks UVB rays but allows UVA rays through. Those UVA rays penetrate your dermis where your blood vessels are located. Researchers have found that UVA rays can break down the vitamin D circulating in your blood vessels. Not only are indoor workers not able to produce vitamin D without exposure to UVB rays, but the vitamin D they do have is at risk of being degraded.

So what is the bottom line? Regular use of sunscreen has *not* been shown to cause vitamin D deficiency but vitamin D deficiency (level < 20 ng/ml) is a significant lifestyle issue for the vast majority of us based on where we live and how we spend our time. I recommend that you have your vitamin D status checked by your health care provider to determine whether you would benefit from increasing dietary sources of vitamin D and/or vitamin D supplementation.

(Note that ranges for *normal* values vary. Conventional medicine ranges are 30 to 50 ng/ml whereas in functional and integrative medicine higher levels ranging from 50 to 80 ng/ml are recommended. There is much discussion about what is the optimal range and I won't insert myself in the middle! I will simply say that you shouldn't supplement blindly. Get tested before you begin supplementing and get retested after three to four months so you can adjust your dosing accordingly. In addition, if you are taking a vitamin D supplementation, adequate potassium and magnesium intake are also required. As with most things, too much of a good thing is not always a good thing.)

If you have dark skin, do you need sunscreen?

The answer is a resounding yes! Melanocytes produce melanin, which is what gives your skin its color. While eumelanin is a type of melanin that provides protection from the sun's UV rays and acts as your body's natural sunscreen, it cannot completely shield your DNA and cells from being damaged. While it is true that individuals with darker skin pigmentation experience less photodamage than individuals with lighter skin and have a lower incidence of skin cancer, due to the greater number, size and distribution of melanin pigment, your skin can still be damaged by the sun's rays. With sun exposure, the skin's natural supply of antioxidants gets quickly depleted. With repeated exposure, cellular and DNA damage occurs. In other words, sunscreen is still an important part of good sun protective habits, even for those with darker skin. Choosing tinted sunscreens may be preferable so that they blend with your skin tone more naturally.

Can you enjoy life outdoors or is it all doom and gloom?

Is it possible to reap the benefits that the sun has to offer, including its warmth, ability to boost your mood, and generate vitamin D? Absolutely, you can! And I encourage you to do so. The caveat is that you need to use caution so you can access the benefits while reducing the risks of being harmed. You now have the knowledge to prepare and protect yourself when you head outside.

Remember, staying safe in the sun is not a pick-and-choose activity. It requires a comprehensive strategy that includes being mindful of the sun's peak intensity, covering up with protective clothing, hats and sunglasses, as well as using sunscreen.

Keep in mind that, although this what you need to protect yourself when you are outdoors, it is not enough. Protecting your skin to maintain your youthful glow begins with how you are nourishing your body every single day and in all aspects of your life. Nourishment provides the foundation for your overall state of health and wellbeing. It encompasses the foods you eat, the products you apply to your skin, the quality of your sleep, how you move your body, your perception of stress, and your relationship with others and most importantly with yourself.

What I've outlined here is akin to the building materials of a house, but just having the supplies is not enough to build the home. You also need a foundation upon which those supplies can be used for construction. If you have superior supplies but a weak foundation, the structure lacks the support it needs and cannot withstand the forces put upon it. That's why, in these pages, I am purposefully not giving you lists of products or creams to apply to your skin. Yes, cleansing, preparing and protecting your skin every morning and every evening is an important part of skin maintenance and rejuvenation, but it needs to be done in conjunction with establishing a strong foundation. You need both to fully thrive.

When you look at your skin and see a sunburn, a tan, an increase in pigmentary changes including moles, wrinkles, changes in skin texture and turgor, your skin is trying to talk to you. It is letting you know it needs you to focus your attention on both your supplies and your foundation. Your body and skin are equipped with an innate supply of antioxidants to satisfy free radicals and the machinery to repair DNA, but the supply and capacity are quickly depleted with environmental exposure, external as well as internal. The good news is you can replenish it. In the remaining chapters, let's explore how you can do just that.

Chapter 4:
NOURISH INSIDE OUT AND OUTSIDE IN

"Let food be thy medicine and medicine be thy food."

Hippocrates

FROM THE INSIDE OUT

Recently, I was out to lunch with a friend, when she commented that today was her "cheat" day. Looking at the menu, she announced she was going to be "bad" and order what she considered a "forbidden" food. As I listened to her dissect the menu into "good" and "bad" foods, my heart ached. I knew all too well that line of thinking — assigning labels to foods and by extension assigning labels to ourselves for eating them.

From my experience, there is no winning in this scenario. The outcome is almost always a feeling of guilt or shame for choosing the "bad" food, or feeling pious for choosing the "good" food (accompanied by a feeling of deprivation that feels bad anyway).

These situations are so pervasive in our society. It's not your fault. With so many diet fads and trends emerging constantly, choosing what to eat can be a source of frustration, anxiety and overwhelm. But it doesn't have to be. Diet is defined as the kinds of food that a person habitually eats. It is a way of eating to nourish your body so it can function optimally, not the more commonly used concept of restriction. So let's block out the media "noise" and dogma that some food is good and other food is bad. There is no room for food shame. It serves no purpose.

What would it look like for you if you saw food as the solution to improving the appearance of your skin, and increasing your energy levels, vitality and mood? How would that change your life? Your relationship to food and eating is the lens through which you nourish your body, so let's work on making it a positive one, shall we? I invite you to join me in shifting your perspective to focus on what you eat in terms of its impact on your health and wellbeing. Nourishing your body is intimately related to the emotions that you have when you do eat. There is no denying it! So instead, let's embrace food and use it to our benefit.

THE APPROACH

How, when and why we eat plays a huge role not only in how we nourish ourselves but also how we nurture ourselves. As you embark on your journey towards better health both physically and emotionally, I want to share with you a reframe that a colleague and mentor shared with me. I wish I knew the original creator to be able to give credit where credit is due, as I find this exercise incredibly powerful in both its simplicity and purpose. The acronym is **HALT** and the intention is to develop an awareness of how you are feeling before you eat. In short, it's a reminder to eat mindfully.

H is for hungry. Before raiding your fridge or pantry, ask yourself, "Am I truly hungry?" The best advice I have ever read was, "Eat for how you want to feel." If you want to feel vibrant, energetic, sexy and kick-ass, then choose foods that will make you feel that way and choose to eat them when you are truly hungry. By taking notice of your motivations, you can decide how to proceed. Remember the labels "good" or "bad" are no longer in your food vocabulary! Be in the moment. Enjoy the texture, the smell, the taste. Savor it.

A is for angry. Are you eating out of anger? If you are, acknowledge it. Don't feel bad about it, but pause. What are you angry about? Is it something that you could address in this moment? Could you use that energy to fuel a walk around the block, a quick jog, jot down what has you so riled up on a piece of paper or call a friend?

L is for lonely. Is feeling alone your reason for seeking comfort in food? Love on someone or something. Your pet, your friends, your family... better yet, love on yourself. Do something that brings a smile to your face. In this time where we're so connected on social media, studies show we feel so *disconnected* from one another in reality; so if you're feeling lonely, know that you are not alone. Acknowledge yourself without judgement and consider what you can do about it.

T is for tired. Are you eating because you are flat-out fatigued or bored? We've all done it, but taking notice of it is the catalyst for change. What could you do instead? Listen to your body. Rest. Ignore the clock. Tune into your body's rhythm.

Feel your body's response to what you eat and drink. Take note of the moments you feel good, reflect on what you put in your body and repeat. Take note of the moments when you feel tired, bloated, and groggy, reflect on what you ingested and minimize or avoid it all together.

THE PREPARATION

Once you have determined that you're hungry and ready to eat, the question turns to how you are eating. Earlier I asked you to take notice if you tend to eat on the go, eat standing up or eat when stressed. Why did I ask you these questions? Because your body's ability to digest, metabolize and assimilate your food is facilitated by the autonomic nervous system.

Your autonomic nervous system is comprised of the sympathetic nervous system, also known as the "fight or flight" response, and the parasympathetic nervous system, referred to as the "rest and digest" response. Depending on how you respond to your environment, your thoughts or your food determines which one of the systems gets "switched on."

Each nervous system has a powerful and essential function.

Your **sympathetic nervous system** switches on when you experience any kind of real or perceived threat. When fear, real or imagined, shows up in your thoughts or environment, for example, being chased by a bear, running late for work, the overflowing to-do list or labeling yourself as "good" or "bad" for indulging in food, you activate your fight-or-flight switch and shift into a stress response. When this happens, your sympathetic nervous system diverts your energy and blood flow away from your digestive tract and sends it to your extremities so you can either fight, flee or freeze in the presence of your stressor. When you are "fighting for your life," digestion takes a backseat on the priority list and the outcome is that your digestion completely shuts down. Although being chased by a bear is an extreme stressor, common stressors like worrying constantly or juggling your kids' activities reduce your ability to digest, assimilate and metabolize your food. Even if your plate is full of healthy food, your body cannot process it properly if it feels under duress.

The good news is that you can optimize your digestive wellness by asserting control on the switch to shift out of the stress response and into rest-and-digest mode by activating your parasympathetic system. Your **parasympathetic nervous system** is your relaxation response; it helps you slow down and recover. When you switch it on, it allows you to conserve your energy by slowing your heart rate, increasing your digestive activity, and helping you take deep, calming breaths.

So how do you help your body keep the parasympathetic nervous system switched on so that you can stay in the rest-and-digest mode?

Here are three strategies to prepare for your meal:

1. ***Sit down and slow down:*** By taking time to sit down to eat and push pause from being on the go constantly and multi-tasking, you can shift out of fight-or-flight mode and into rest-and-digest mode. It will also allow you to chew your food thoroughly and completely so your body has the best chance of absorbing the nutrients you are consuming.

2. ***Breathe:*** Take a deep breath — fully, slowly, deeply — with the intention of relaxing and being fully present at the dining table. Your breath is intimately connected to your mood and emotions. Have you noticed how quickly you breathe when you're stressed out? Well, the fastest way to relax is to slow your breathing.

3. ***Savor the flavor:*** Activate all your senses by enjoying the food on your plate. Take notice of the smell, texture, and taste. Tuning into how you good you feel while you eat will turn on your parasympathetic nervous system.

THE PROCESS

You may have heard the old adage "you are what you eat," but in actuality you are what your bacteria eat. Now that you're relaxed and ready to eat, the next part is keeping your gut health on track so you can reap the benefits of the nutrients you are consuming.

Hippocrates said, "All disease begins in the gut." With 70% of your immune cells housed in the walls of your gut, it makes sense that your gut health plays a significant role in your overall health. Your gut is lined with trillions of bacteria known as your gut microbiome, which helps your body with nearly every function, including digesting your food, thinking clearly, maintaining a healthy weight, and supporting a healthy complexion.

When your gut microbiome is in balance, you stay healthy, have lots of energy and experience stable moods. When your gut microbiome is out of balance, there is an increase in inflammation and permeability of the intestinal lining (referred to as "leaky gut"). The role of your intestinal lining is to serve as a strong barrier between your gut and the rest of your body. When your intestinal wall becomes leaky, particles of food enter your bloodstream, triggering your immune system to attack them, and ultimately your own tissues. This leads to inflammation, food sensitivities and allergies as well as autoimmunity. An imbalance in your gut microbiome also causes an abnormal growth of gut bacteria called dysbiosis. Dysbiosis in the microbiome has been associated with numerous diseases, including inflammatory bowel disease, multiple sclerosis, diabetes, allergies, asthma, autism and cancer, as well as skin issues including acne, rosacea, eczema and psoriasis.

Unfortunately, an unbalanced gut microbiome or dysbiosis has become a common problem for many of us. Diets high in processed foods and sugar, consuming conventionally raised meat and dairy products full of hormones, rounds of antibiotics and chronic stress have been tagged as major contributing factors. Evidence for the impact of stress on the gut microbiome dates back to over 70 years ago when dermatologists Drs. Stokes and Pillsbury linked emotional states including depression, worry and anxiety to an alteration in the gut microbiome leading to skin conditions including hives, acne and skin inflammation.

Even if your microbiome is currently out of balance, the great news is that you have the power to change it! The bacteria in your gut is incredibly responsive to the foods you eat. In a recent study, researcher Lawrence David found that within just a few days not only was there a variation in the abundance of different kinds of bacteria in the gut, but also the kinds of genes they were expressing. This is exciting! It means you can begin to change your microbiome with every meal to improve your gut health, and in turn your skin health.

THE PLAN

So now you know that your gut microbiome responds to what you feed it, what should you eat to achieve youthful, radiant looking skin that is more UV-resistant? Simple: whole, unprocessed nutrient-dense foods that are low in sugar, anti-inflammatory and rich in antioxidants. Paired with a curated selection of supplements, your body and your skin will thank you.

Let's look at why:

1. **Foods low in sugar:** In Chapter 2, I shared the ways in which sugar wreaks havoc on your body and skin through the formation of AGEs and inflammation. AGEs not only interfere with your collagen's function but also lead to its destruction, contributing to wrinkles, sagging, dryness,

The Skin Whisperer

irritation and a sallow complexion. Foods high in sugar as well as foods that are more readily converted to glucose (especially refined carbohydrate-rich foods like white bread, pasta and rice) are referred to as high glycemic foods. A diet largely featuring high glycemic foods creates glucose quickly, which can cause a blood sugar spike followed by an insulin spike. This, in turn, can cause cellular inflammation, especially if you eat a lot of them. Over time, consumption of a high glycemic diet contributes to insulin resistance, which is linked to skin aging and worsening of acne, rosacea, psoriasis, and eczema.

In the world of nutrition, there are two terms used that can help you gauge the sugar impact of your food. By understanding how the foods you eat impact blood sugar, you can choose foods that promote slower digestion, a more gradual release of sugar into the bloodstream and a more steady release of insulin rather than spikes. Your blood sugar and insulin levels stay nice and even — no rollercoaster — and that's what you want. These terms are **glycemic index** and **glycemic load**.

Glycemic index (GI) is a value given to foods based on how slowly or quickly those foods cause an increase in blood sugar levels. Food low on the GI scale releases glucose steadily and slowly. Foods high on the GI releases glucose quickly. It's important to note that not all foods are created equal as two different foods with the same amount of carbohydrate can have different GI numbers. The smaller the number, the less the food impacts your blood sugar.

- 55 or less = low
- 56-69 = medium
- 70 or higher = high

For example, pure glucose has a GI of 100, ice cream 62, and an apple is 36. In this context, consistently choosing foods in the lowest categories is your best bet. It's worth noting that GI can be affected by how a food is prepared, its ripeness and with which foods it is paired. This is why incorporating fat, fiber and protein into all your meals and snacks is recommended, to help decrease overall GI of a meal. So put some almond butter on your whole grain toast and sprinkle flax meal into your cereal. (Choose gluten-free varieties if you notice you aren't tolerating gluten-containing foods.)

GI is only part of the blood sugar story, however. That's where glycemic load (GL) comes into play. GL tells you how quickly the food makes glucose enter your bloodstream *and* how much glucose it delivers. GL tells you the real-life impact of a food on your blood sugar.

By choosing foods that have a low glycemic index and a low glycemic load, you can reduce the amount of sugar and insulin released into your bloodstream. You can avoid the blood sugar-insulin rollercoaster and keep your energy levels, mood and inflammatory response well balanced. Some packaged foods may have GI listed, but since we are all about whole foods, checking out glycemic index and glycemic load lists on the internet is your best bet. Harvard University has one with more than 100 foods listed.

2. **Anti-inflammatory foods:** You are now familiar with the role of sugar in inflammation. Hopefully, I've convinced you to rethink your relationship with it. Another big contributor to inflammation is trans fats. Although there is naturally occurring trans fat in some meat and dairy products, the vast majority is derived through an industrial process that adds hydrogen to vegetable oil, which

causes the oil to become solid at room temperature. This partially hydrogenated oil is commonly used in fast fried foods and processed foods, because it is less likely to spoil and inexpensive to make.

The FDA has determined these fats to be unsafe. Here's why. Trans fat raises your "harmful" (LDL) cholesterol and lowers your "helpful" (HDL) cholesterol, increasing your risk of stroke, heart attack and diabetes. More importantly, trans fats are pro-inflammatory. As chronic inflammation has been found to be the culprit of aging skin as well as a host of diseases including autoimmune and Alzheimer's disease, it drives home the point that the foods you choose can have a significant impact on the health of your skin, your body and your microbiome. Avoiding trans fats will do your body and skin good.

Other foods that are known to be pro-inflammatory for many people include gluten, dairy, corn, eggs, soy, shellfish, preservatives and additives, especially dyes. Take notice of how you feel when you consume these items. Do you feel bloated, tired, wired, irritable, anxious or break out in a rash? If you answered yes to any of these, you may consider keeping a journal to try to tease out what your triggers may be, which will enable you to eliminate them.

3. **Food rich in antioxidants:** In Chapter 2, I shared that free radicals are created as part of your body's natural metabolism, and to an even greater degree when your body is under stress. You are also affected by them as a result of exposure to pollution, chemicals and sunlight. Free radicals cause damage to your skin and body when they steal electrons from your healthy cells as a means to regain their molecules' stability. Think of them as a villain to your skin. Antioxidants are your body's superheroes, because

they donate electrons to the free radicals, neutralizing their ability to scavenge and cause damage. Because UV exposure and other environmental factors can quickly deplete your skin's innate antioxidant reserve, it cannot handle the amount of free radicals, cellular and DNA damage that is created. The result is premature skin aging, and suppression of the immune system with subsequent risk of developing melanoma and NMSC.

Eating foods and using topical products on your skin that are rich in antioxidants can increase the antioxidant capacity of your bloodstream and tissues to have greater protection from the sun, aging and inflammation.

Before we dive into the specifics of beneficial foods, I want to share some basics that will serve you well no matter what genre of cuisine or way of eating you prefer. And let me be clear, there is no "perfect" way of eating. There are so many options out there, whether you gravitate towards paleo, ketogenic, Whole 30, Mediterranean, vegan, vegetarian or the umpteen other trends on the market. The bottom line is this: focus on **adequate hydration**, choose **whole foods** from the cleanest source you can (ideally organic), and incorporate **fat, fiber and protein** into every meal.

Avoid overeating

Eat to feel satiated rather than stuffed. Overeating causes insulin resistance and contributes to oxidative stress, which you now know creates significant issues for your skin and your overall health. When I lived in Okinawa, Japan, an island famous for longevity and vitality, I learned and adapted their cultural habit called **hara hachi bu**, which means eat only until you are 80% full. Of course, there's no way to know exactly how full you are, but it's a general guideline. Since our brains are about 10 to 20 minutes behind our stomachs, usually when you think you're 80% full, you're actually full. When we eat to 100% full, we are usually overstuffing ourselves. Play with this and take notice of how you feel.

What about hydration?

Think of water as the elixir of life, as every cell and every system in your body needs it to survive. Your body is composed of about 60% water and this composition needs to be maintained for optimal health. Drinking water helps you balance your body fluids, which are required to aid digestion, absorption, circulation, transportation of nutrients, regulation of body temperature and creation of saliva. Water also helps keep your joints lubricated, prevents infections and helps your kidney and liver rid your body of toxins.

Your body loses large quantities of water every day through respiration, perspiration and elimination (urination and bowel movements). This needs to be replaced by drinking water as well as consuming foods that contain a higher water content.

In addition to water loss, you are losing electrolytes including sodium and potassium. When you are not adequately hydrated, your organs cannot function properly or at their best. A lack of hydration can contribute to impaired brain function and memory, headaches, constipation, muscle fatigue, weight gain and diminished athletic performance. It can also impact your skin.

Skin cells, like every other cell in your body, are made up water. If your skin is not getting enough water, the lack of hydration will show up as a dry, tight and flaky appearance. Your hair may also feel dry and brittle if you are not consuming enough water. Dry skin has less resilience and will be prone to wrinkling and fine lines. Hydrating your skin is an inside and outside job; you need to drink water as well as help your skin retain hydration by using moisturizer especially after you get out of the shower to seal that water in.

So how much should you drink? The recommendation is to consume about half your body weight in ounces of water per day, which should average out to be around 8 to 12 cups. Your needs may increase depending on how physically active you are or if you are in a warmer climate and need to replenish your resources from excessive sweating. You may also consider adding electrolytes to your water in those circumstances. You may also need to boost your intake if you consume caffeine and alcohol, which draws water out of your cells.

Simply put: drink more water. I know it's not always the most appealing beverage, but it doesn't have to be boring. Jazz it up by adding frozen berries, a splash of lemon, lime or watermelon. My advice: ditch the plastic water bottles and use glass or stainless steel instead. Although your plastic may be labeled BPA-free, manufacturers have substituted BPA for a close cousin that can leach chemicals into your water supply just the same, so avoid it altogether when you can. Use this as an excuse to go get yourself a super fun or cute water bottle that you can't resist using!

Why eat whole food?
- Whole food is real food. It's food in its most natural state. Your body knows how to process, break down and use real food as energy. They are easier for your body to digest.
- Whole foods are nutrient-dense. Per bite, you get more actual nutrition and nourishing necessities for your body.
- Whole foods usually have minimal labeling or packaging. If the food does have a label, read it. The fewer ingredients the better. It should have everything that you (and/or your

kids) can pronounce. If you have no idea what an ingredient on the label is because it's some long chemical-sounding word, put it back on the shelf. Whole foods do not contain chemicals, artificial preservatives or sweeteners.

- Whole foods are quality fuel for your body. And quality fuel = higher efficiency = mood stabilizing = happier you.

Why eat fat, fiber and protein with every meal?

To balance your blood sugar, experience satiety and have energy throughout your day, create snacks and meals that combine this trifecta. Meals with a mix of fat, fiber and protein are digested at a slower pace, avoiding insulin spikes and supporting a more even absorption of glucose, which in turn keeps your blood sugar levels balanced and helps you feel full longer. Feeling fuller for longer will kick to the curb those hunger and sugar cravings associated with blood sugar crashes. There are no hard and fast rules regarding the proportion of fat, fiber and protein. You are unique and your needs are going to be different from those of others. Remember, this is about eating for how you want to feel, so experiment with different proportions and combinations, and take notice of how you feel after each meal.

Fat

Gone are the days where fat is your foe. Healthy fats are your friends because every cell in your body uses fatty acids to build and maintain itself. Fat is important for absorption of vitamins A, D, E and K needed for glowing skin. What's more: you need to consume essential fatty acids (like omega-3), because your body can't make them, nor survive without them! Your body needs fatty acids to help balance your hormones and blood sugar, create and maintain healthy cell membranes and the energy within your cells, support your brain's ability to focus and function, and manage inflammation. Essential fatty acids are vital for healthy skin because they help cells retain water, so a diet rich in them can help to minimize the appearance of aging, cellulite and oily skin. Below I'll share foods that provide good sources of fat.

Fiber

Incorporating fiber into your meals — from whole grains, legumes, vegetables, fruits, nuts and seeds — is vital for your gut to function properly. Not only does fiber help keep you feeling fuller for longer, it makes bowel movements easier, helps remove bad bacteria from the colon, feeds the good bacteria in the colon and facilitates removal of toxins. When adding fiber to your diet, both soluble and insoluble types, go slowly to see how you feel and be sure to maintain your hydration. Adding too much fiber too soon has the potential to speed up elimination for some or cause bloating and discomfort for others, so listen to your body and adjust as necessary.

Protein

It doesn't matter whether you choose animal or plant sources for your protein. What matters is that you incorporate it into your meals and snacks. Protein provides amino acids, which are the building blocks for every cell of every organ in your body. You need protein to help your body repair, recover, grow and develop. Simply put: you need protein to survive and thrive. The amount of protein you need is also individual, so experiment with that as well as with different sources. For animal sources, I recommend organic and grass-fed meat or dairy whenever possible. For plant sources, I suggest organic; ideally sprouted when feasible.

The recommendations that follow have features of the Mediterranean diet, which is based on fruits, vegetables, mono-unsaturated fats like those found in olive oil and a healthy ratio of omega-3 to omega-6 polyunsaturated fatty acids. Eating foods rich in these compounds is associated with increased longevity and overall good health, including protecting against cancer and heart disease. Best of all, there is evidence that these nutrients help prevent skin cancer specifically! So let's dig in!

PROTECTION FROM THE INSIDE OUT: THE FOOD
Foods rich in vitamin C:

Vitamin C or ascorbic acid fights free radicals, increases immunity and is essential for the production of collagen and elastin. This is why vitamin C is so good for your skin, whether you eat it or apply it topically. As a water-soluble vitamin, your body quickly excretes vitamin C rather than storing it, so consuming vitamin-C-rich foods daily is recommended.

By neutralizing free radicals caused by ultraviolet light and increasing the production of collagen and elastin, vitamin C has been found to decrease sunburns due to UVB, promote skin cell renewal, reduce fine lines and wrinkles, lighten and even skin tones, and maintain youthful skin resilience. In other words, vitamin C plays an essential role in inhibiting skin aging. A split-face study showed that topical application of vitamin C decreased the appearance of pigmentation, inflammation, wrinkling and dehydration of facial skin compared to the untreated side after 12 weeks.

There is an abundance of foods to choose from to get your vitamin C. As it degrades quickly with cooking, eating foods fresh and raw to obtain this vitamin is your best bet to maximize the benefits.

So where do you find it? These are some great sources:

- pomegranate
- cantaloupe
- collards
- strawberries
- kale
- mangoes
- onions
- oranges
- pineapples
- spinach
- tomatoes
- green peas
- currants
- raspberries
- Brussels sprouts
- cauliflower
- cabbage

As a side note, you'll notice I didn't emphasize citrus as your primary source of vitamin C. I'm a big fan of lemons, limes and oranges, but when it comes to sun protection, I favor other foods to boost your antioxidant reserve. Here's why. Citrus contains psoralens, a chemical that makes your skin more sensitive to the sun. A study in the Journal of Clinical Oncology highlighted a correlation between consumption of citrus and an increased risk of skin cancers, both basal cell and squamous cell. Another study found an increased risk of melanoma. The highest incidence of skin cancer was found with the highest consumption of citrus fruit, especially grapefruit, which has the highest level of psoralens. So enjoy your citrus fruit, but especially when heading outdoors, protect your skin. Get all the benefits and minimize your risks!

Foods rich in vitamin E:

Vitamin E or tocopherol is an antioxidant that plays many roles. It has potent anti-inflammatory effects and improves the ability of your skin and vessels to act as protective barriers, improve healing, and reduce scarring. It also plays a role in making your DNA. Similar to vitamin C, vitamin E neutralizes free radicals preventing cell damage, and helping to prevent skin cancer and skin aging. A study in the Journal of Investigative Dermatology highlighted the synergistic effects of taking vitamin C and E supplementation to reduce sunburns and protect against DNA damage. This is the reason these vitamins have become staples in skincare products in the marketplace.

It's worthwhile to note that vitamin E supplements may cause side effects, including bruising and bleeding problems, so always check in with your physician to see if supplementation is appropriate for you. Vitamin E is fat soluble, which means your body can store it in fat. Unlike vitamin C, therefore, it's not as important to eat vitamin E every day.

Where to find it? Great sources of vitamin E include:

- avocados
- dark-green leafy vegetables

- anchovies
- salmon
- nuts
- seeds
- carrots
- butternut squash
- sweet potatoes
- pumpkin
- olive oil
- eggs
- organ meats

Foods rich in vitamin A:

Vitamin A packs a powerful punch as an antioxidant, whether it's eaten or used topically. It plays an important role in the maintenance and repair of skin tissue, boosts immunity, slows the aging process, neutralizes free radicals, and helps block the formation of cancer.

Vitamin A, also referred to as retinoids, is actually a group of biologically active compounds found naturally in plant and animal tissues. Animal sources of vitamin A are fat-soluble and in the form of retinoic acid, retinal and retinol. Because they are stored in our tissues, too much animal-derived vitamin A can build up in the body and become toxic. This is the reason why supplements and drugs with vitamin A are not recommended for pregnant women.

In contrast, plant sources of vitamin A are water-soluble and don't accumulate in the body, so toxicity is rare. The caveat is that vitamin A in fruits and vegetables in a precursor form known as carotenoids has to be converted in the body into a usable retinoid form. There are several subsets of carotenoids that work together to provide health benefits to our bodies. Beta-carotene is one of the carotenoids that the body can convert into a usable form of vitamin A. Yellow and orange fruits and vegetables like carrots and sweet potatoes are rich in beta-carotene. The skin benefits of beta-carotene are an increase in the production of collagen and glycosaminoglycans, which improve the integrity of skin and help it retain moisture to prevent flaking, dryness and scaling. What's more: an increased beta-carotene intake has been associated with a decreased risk of melanoma, according to a retrospective dietary analysis in a control study of melanoma patients. In a placebo-controlled clinical study, sunburn intensity after UV exposure was lower in subjects receiving carotenoid supplements.

The best way to get the benefits of retinoids and beta-carotene is from your diet, good sources being:

- carrots
- squash
- sweet potatoes
- cantaloupe
- apricots
- mangoes
- eggs
- shrimp
- fish (tuna, trout, salmon)

- shrimp
- liver
- milk

Although I just claimed eating your antioxidants is best, I have to say that using topical vitamin A on your skin in its various forms including tretinoin (prescription only) and retinol (non-prescription) has a profound impact when it comes to skin cancer prevention and skin aging. Before you head to the drug store, here's what you need to know: topical retinoid products come in different concentrations and strengths, which can influence the degree to which they can cause dryness, irritation and increased sun sensitivity, which is why they are only to be used at night followed by strict use of sun protection, including sunscreen, during the day. When in doubt of what product to use or if you are interested in a prescription strength topical retinoid consult your dermatologist. As a general rule for use, a little goes a long way. The key is to start gradually and with a small amount, typically a dollop the size of a green pea that you divide evenly and rub into your forehead, cheeks, nose and chin. If you know you have a tendency toward sensitive skin, start with a smaller amount and do not use every night. Instead, begin to use the product every other night or every three nights. If you find your skin becomes too dry, flaky, red or inflamed you may have to decrease the frequency to only once or twice weekly. Should your entire face become red, inflamed and irritated, you may need a lower concentration or strength. It's also possible you are unable to tolerate use. Again, when in doubt, consult with your dermatologist.

Despite the need for caution, I am a raving fan, because studies have shown that topical vitamin A increases collagen production, prevents collagen breakdown, exfoliates skin, increases skin cell turnover, decreases melanin production, and evens out tone, texture and moisture levels of skin. Bottom line: it has profound effects in reversing sun damage, diminishing skin aging and improving acne. You get some serious bang for your buck using topical retinoids!

Foods rich in carotenoids:

There are several different kinds of carotenoids — like lycopene, lutein and zeaxanthin — that do not convert to vitamin A like beta-carotene does. Yet they have potent antioxidant and anti-inflammatory effects. In fact, lycopene found in red fruits and vegetables like tomatoes, watermelon and guava is celebrated as the most powerful antioxidant measured in food. Lycopene is especially powerful in protecting the skin. A study in the British Journal of Dermatology showed that after 10 weeks, women who regularly ate tomato paste compared to those who didn't were 40% less likely to be sunburned. Lycopene is fat soluble, so add some olive oil to your tomato sauce to boost the benefits and increase your absorption.

The carotenoids lutein and zeaxanthin have also been shown to help protect the skin from UV exposure. These antioxidants are essential to eye health, as they filter out harmful wavelengths and act to neutralize free radicals. Lutein and zeaxanthin are also found in your skin where they help prevent damage and maintain the structural integrity of your skin.

Where can we find the best sources of carotenoids? They are most abundant in cooked green leafy vegetables like:

- romaine lettuce
- spinach

- Swiss chard
- kale
- collard greens
- mustard greens
- turnip greens

All of these foods contain beta-carotene as well as lutein and zeaxanthin.

Foods rich in polyphenols:

Polyphenols possess anti-inflammatory, immunomodulatory and antioxidant properties, which is why they are considered among the most promising group of compounds to be researched and implemented as an ideal cancer-prevention strategy.

The majority of natural polyphenols are pigments — including yellow, red or purple — and can absorb UV radiation. Polyphenols can absorb the entire UVB spectrum of wavelengths as well as part of the UVA and UVC spectra. What does this mean? It means polyphenols can prevent penetration of UV radiation into the skin and may act as a sunscreen to reduce inflammation, oxidative stress and the DNA-damaging effects of UV radiation in the skin. This is why eating foods rich in polyphenols provides benefit. It's also why polyphenols have been incorporated into topical skincare products recently.

Among foods rich in polyphenols that pack a powerful skin-protective punch are deeply colored fruits and cruciferous vegetables. Think:

- watercress
- arugula
- bok choy
- broccoli
- Brussels sprouts
- kale
- pomegranate
- blackcurrants
- grapes
- plums
- cherries
- strawberries

These vegetables supply phytochemicals such as indoles that help stop cancer before it starts. They block enzymes that activate carcinogens as well as helping prevent and repair DNA damage that can lead to cancer. An Italian study showed that eating vegetables more than five times a week, with dark green and cruciferous vegetables at the top of the list, decreased the risk of melanoma. Among the fruits, pomegranate has been found to have such significant health benefits, it has been dubbed, "nature's power fruit" because of its strong antioxidant and anti-inflammatory properties as well as its high levels of vitamin C (provides about 40% of the daily requirement). Studies have shown that pomegranate-derived products either consumed or applied topically protect against UV-induced oxidative stress, cell death and cancer formation. In other words, this "power fruit" has shown promise against photoaging as well as skin cancer formation and progression. So fill up your plate!

Foods rich in healthy fats:

Specifically here, I'm talking about omega-3 fatty acid and olive oil.

Omega-3 fatty acid is a polyunsaturated fat. There are three main omega-3s: eicosapentaenoic acid (EPA) and docosahexaenoic acid (DHA), found in cold-water fish including salmon, sardines and albacore tuna; and alpha-linolenic acid (ALA), found in flaxseed, soybean oil, walnuts and pumpkin seeds.

Although your body cannot make its own ALA, which means you have to obtain it through your diet, your body is quite proficient at converting ALA to EPA and DHA, the forms your body *can* use. Omega-3 fatty acids help keep skin healthy, looking younger and less wrinkled by maintaining its natural oil barrier. Even though omega-3 fatty acids don't have antioxidant properties, they fight free radical damage and exert significant anti-inflammatory effects by blocking a chemical that promotes skin cancer progression. As inflammation is a major contributor to all disease, including skin cancer, acne, rosacea, and psoriasis, eating omega-3 fatty acids several times a week is recommended. If you aren't a fish lover, you can supplement with flaxseed oil or oral supplementation of 1000 mg a day.

Here are some great sources of omega-3 fatty acids including ALA, EPA and DHA:

- wild caught salmon
- sardines

- albacore tuna
- oysters
- mackerel
- flaxseed oil or freshly ground
- grass-fed beef
- seaweed
- hemp seed oil
- walnuts
- chia seeds
- egg yolks
- herring

Extra virgin olive oil is a mono-unsaturated fat and a key component of the Mediterranean diet. Olive oil is rich in at least 30 phenolic acid antioxidants including squalene and oleic acid, which have been shown to protect against skin cancer and aging by inhibiting oxidative stress. A clinical study suggested that olive oil should afford considerable protection against not only photo-aging and skin cancer, but also breast and colon cancer by inhibiting cellular oxidative damage.

Foods rich in zinc, copper and selenium:

These minerals are involved in destroying free radicals, boosting the immune system and reducing the risk of cancer. Selenium has anti-aging and anti-inflammatory properties, while zinc increases the level of proteins involved in DNA repair and reduces the kind of DNA damage that contributes to cancer formation. Copper is vital to the formation of collagen and elastin, and skin regeneration.

Foods rich in zinc include:

- grass-fed beef
- lamb
- chickpeas
- lentils
- black beans

You can find selenium in:

- yellowfin tuna
- sardines
- halibut
- brazil nuts
- chicken
- eggs
- spinach

Copper-rich foods include:

- dried apricots
- dark chocolate
- almonds
- lentils
- asparagus

Beverages rich in antioxidants: tea and coffee

Tea has been consumed as a popular beverage worldwide for thousands of years because of its health benefits. Studies show that drinking green and black tea can help prevent skin cancer, though the evidence is stronger for green tea. Green tea contains polyphenols, the plant chemicals with powerful antioxidant, anti-inflammatory and tumor-inhibiting properties. The polyphenols in green tea have been found to prevent DNA damage from UV radiation, repair DNA damage, prevent the progression of DNA damage to cancer and fend off UV-induced immunosuppression allowing cancer to grow. Studies have shown green tea either consumed or applied directly to the skin topically prior to sun exposure has helped protect against sunburn as well as prevent UVB-induced depletion of antioxidant enzyme levels required to fend off DNA damage. What's more: an Italian study showed that frequent green tea consumption was protective against melanoma. The benefits were realized from drinking four to six freshly brewed cups a day, so drink up!

Coffee is rich in antioxidants, including flavonoids and polyphenols. Studies have shown that higher consumption of caffeinated coffee was associated with lower risk for basal cell carcinoma and may also have an effect at lowering the risk of melanoma as well. In a clinical study of over 90,000 Caucasian women, it was found that those who drank six or more cups of coffee per day, had a 30% decrease in prevalence of non-melanoma skin cancer. In a separate study, coffee consumption of one cup per day was associated with a 3% reduction in melanoma risk, while another study showed a 20% decreased prevalence of malignant melanoma consuming four cups a day. The sweet spot may turn out to be somewhere in the middle but more research needs to be done. For now though, we know that the benefit is tied to the bioactive chemicals in coffee, including caffeine and chlorogenic acid, so don't switch to decaf just yet!

Furthermore, coffee may protect skin against damage from ultraviolet light through its roasting process, which generates vitamin B3 (nicotinic acid) and nicotinamide. These have been shown to suppress UVB-induced skin damage.

Seasonings with benefits:

There are numerous herbs and spices that possess powerful antioxidant and anti-aging properties. Among those common to Mediterranean cooking are:

- oregano
- rosemary
- parsley
- sage
- dill
- coriander
- thyme
- bay leaf
- cinnamon
- basil
- star anise
- celery seed
- curry powder

Parsley contains a compound called apigenin, which helps protect the skin from the sun. Rosemary contains carnosol, which has been shown to have anti-cancer properties.

Other spices including turmeric, ginger and garlic are especially powerful anti-inflammatory agents that not only improve the appearance of skin, but also have sun-protective benefits. In the lab, they have been shown to inhibit skin cancer formation. Turmeric inhibits UV-induced cellular damage, reduces inflammation, and prevents cellular changes leading to tumor formation. So find any excuse to add these flavors in.

Sweets that just got sweeter:

In case you need another reason to eat it, researchers have found that dark chocolate is rich in flavanols, which are potent antioxidants that help your skin protect itself from UV damage, fight free radicals and increase blood flow. In one study, flavanols in dark chocolate even improved skin hydration and thickness — both super important for younger looking skin. You only reap the benefit by eating chocolate with a cocoa percentage of 70% or higher, but when you do, you can say goodbye to wrinkles, sunburn and sun spots, and welcome a radiant glow.

THE SUPPLEMENTS

While I believe food trumps supplements all day long, our food sources may not offer the level of nutrients we need to maintain optimal wellness and skin health. The following are supplements that have been shown to be beneficial for keeping your skin looking younger as well as protected in the sun. Before taking any supplements, research for the best quality, and check in with your physician to make sure they are appropriate for you.

Astaxanthin is a carotenoid and comes from microalgae in the Arctic marine environment. Considered to be the most potent carotenoid, it is 10 times as potent as beta-carotene and 100 times stronger than vitamin E in its anti-inflammatory capabilities. It has been shown to protect against UVA-induced DNA damage. Salmon, crab, lobster and shrimp get their red color from eating an astaxanthin-rich algae diet.

Vitamins E and C are abundant in food, so filling your plate is the optimal way to get your supply. That said, I recommend using these antioxidants topically on your skin every day to improve the tone and texture of your skin. This way you can ensure both your inside and outside are getting the nourishment you need. These antioxidants help prevent free radicals from forming during UV exposure, improve the skin's protective barrier, and have anti-inflammatory effects. Vitamin C plays an important role in the synthesis of collagen and elastin, and vitamin E plays a role in preventing collagen breakdown.

Resveratrol is a naturally occurring polyphenolic compound found in grapes, red wine, some berries, and peanuts. Although the benefits associated with resveratrol are significant — including anti-aging, sun protection, reducing inflammation and cancer prevention — a challenge with resveratrol is its bioavailability. It is rapidly metabolized meaning it disappears from the bloodstream very quickly. Although I am big fan of red wine, the best bang for your buck with this antioxidant is using it topically.

Vitamin D, as I shared in Chapter 3, is vital to our health with almost every cell in our body in possession of a vitamin D receptor. Celebrated for its bone-building and immune-boosting benefits, vitamin D is essential for normal skin cell metabolism, growth, repair and maintaining the barrier function of the skin. In fact, formulations of topical vitamin D are used to help manage skin conditions like psoriasis. Vitamin D boosts the skin's immune system and helps destroy free radicals, highlighting its anti-aging benefit. Research on vitamin D supplementation for skin cancer prevention as well as supplemental therapy for managing melanoma makes understanding your current vitamin D levels a top priority. Ask your physician to check your levels to help you best determine what oral supplementation support you may need to optimize the health of your skin, bones and immune function. The daily recommendation is 600 IU but this is likely not enough for your individual needs.

Niacinamide, AKA nicotinamide, in both its oral and topical forms, is a type of vitamin B3 and has proven to have beneficial effects in acne, rosacea, atopic dermatitis and now skin cancer. When UV hits the skin, it can suppress the immune system and damage DNA. When DNA damage exceeds our skin's ability to repair it, premature skin aging and skin cancers develop. By recharging the skin's energy supplies when they are depleted from making these repairs, nicotinamide not only boosts the immune system's ability to repair DNA, but also reduces UV-induced immunosuppression. Several studies by Damian and colleagues have shown that 500 mg of nicotinamide taken twice daily reduces the rate of new skin pre-cancers (actinic keratosis), basal cell carcinomas and squamous cell carcinomas by 23% in patients with a previous history of NMSC. Her research also suggests that nicotinamide may provide similar benefits to melanoma. The jury is still out on whether these benefits translate to people who have never had NMSC.

Polypodium leucotomas (PL) is derived from a tropical fern grown in Central and South America, and is a key ingredient in several oral dietary supplements currently on the market. PL offers sun protective benefits as an antioxidant with anti-inflammatory, chemoprotective and immunomodulatory effects. The antioxidant activity of PL is primarily driven by its rich source of phenolic acids, including caffeic acid and ferulic acid. As an antioxidant, PL boosts the ability of our body's own antioxidant systems to help prevent sunburn, neutralize free radicals, inhibit DNA damage and UV-induced inflammation, and upregulate a molecule to suppress tumor formation. A recent study showed that a dose of 240 mg taken twice daily suppressed sunburn and extended the time outdoors before tanning occurred in the skin. These findings suggest that PL offers the potential to be an excellent adjunct to other sun protective measures.

FROM THE OUTSIDE IN

Hopefully, you now have a better understanding of the importance of eating a wide variety of foods to get your healthy dose of vitamins, minerals and antioxidants. What you eat or don't eat can show up on your skin. For example, not having enough fat in your diet can cause skin inflammation, increased susceptibility to skin infection, hair loss and scaling. Similarly, not having enough protein in your diet can show up as poor wound healing, hair thinning and grooves in your nails.

We have touched on the benefit of using topical vitamins for diminishing the effects of sun damage, including vitamin C, vitamin E, vitamin B3 and topical retinoids. But one of the keys to nourishing your skin from the outside in is paying attention to the products you use and the ingredients they contain to achieve the benefits.

In healthy skin, the surface of the epidermis is covered by a thin slightly acidic film called the acid mantle with a pH that ranges between 4.5 and 5.5. The film is maintained by the oily secretions from the sebaceous glands (sebum), the salty and watery mixture from the eccrine sweat glands and secretions from normal skin flora (microbiome). The acid mantle is both a physical and chemical barrier and serves as the skin's first line of defense. It prevents dehydration, protects against environmental pollutants, and maintains pH balance so skin stays supple, smooth and vibrant. It also prevents harmful bacteria, fungi and viruses from invading the skin which flourish in an alkaline (basic) pH.

When skin is healthy the cells in the stratum corneum are arranged like a brick wall. They are neatly stacked and held together by "mortar" which are intercellular connections and epidermal lipids (fats). These fats, which include ceramides, cholesterol and fatty acids, paired with keratinocyte derived Natural Moisturizing Factor, are essential to create your skin's protective barrier and bind in moisture. They protect your skin from damage, aid in your skin's repair and keep dirt and environmental chemicals out. When the skin pH is elevated to become more alkaline or "the mortar" (lipids) are missing, the skin can become dry, rough, itchy, sensitive and red associated with barrier damage. By altering the pH, it also renders the skin vulnerable to invasion by harmful bugs which crave the higher alkaline pH.

Skin health is also influenced by over one trillion bacteria on our skin, originating from over 1000 species, comprising the skin microbiome. The skin microbiome joins the gut microbiome in playing a significant role in your health. The diversity of bacteria varies by location on the body, whether the location is dry, moist, oily or hairy, the amount of light present and pH levels. The skin microbiome helps keep skin plump and firm, supports wound healing, and a recent study in Frontiers in Microbiology has suggested it may play a role skin cancer prevention by guarding against oxidative stress and free radicals. A healthy skin microbiome not only prefers a relatively acidic pH, it helps create and maintain it with a pH around 5, which is in sync with the acid mantle for providing an optimal moisture barrier and protection from infection. What's more is that these helpful bugs communicate with your immune system to upregulate it to release antimicrobial peptides to ward off harmful bugs as well as downregulate it to help soothe inflammation.

When your skin microbiome is in balance, your complexion glows. When your skin microbiome is out of balance, due to diet, sun exposure, environmental pollutants, and skin care products, there is an increase in inflammation and permeability of the skin barrier. When your skin barrier is disrupted it can result in skin sensitivity, breakouts and flares of eczema, rosacea and psoriasis.

Harsh ingredients in skin care products can contribute to dysbiosis of your skin microbiome, alter skin pH and strip the skin of its essential lipids ("mortar"). Washing the skin with moderately or highly alkaline soap or detergents both disrupts the microbiome as well as strips the acid mantle. Over-exfoliating with aggressive scrubs or using a face brush too often can weaken your skin's defense system. Products like foaming cleanser can dry out the skin and toners can alter the skin pH, stripping away the acid mantle and further exacerbate sensitive skin. Although active ingredients like glycolic or salicylic acids are beneficial for exfoliation and maintaining the acid mantle, they can make matters worse if you already have dry and irritated skin.

Choosing products that both attract and bind water, known as humectants as well as seal in moisture, known as occlusive agents are better options to heal the skin. Examples of humectants include glycerin, hyaluronic acid and aloe vera and examples of occlusive agents include shea butter, jojoba oil and lanolin. Petrolatum (Petroleum jelly), derived from highly refined crude oil, is a well known and effective occlusive agent though recent controversy over its safety regarding contamination with polyaromatic hydrocarbons has caused it to fall out of favor in some circles. Although no studies have ever shown a direct link between petrolatum and cancer, the Environmental Working Group ranks it as a moderate hazard and the European Union put numerous grades of petrolatum on a list of dangerous substances. That said, there are plenty of alternative occlusive agents on the market and I personally choose to use these in as many products as I can.

By now, you can appreciate that the products you use on the skin surface can significantly impact the integrity of your skin structure, function and microbiome.

Along these lines, just as we feed our body with nourishing food, we need to feed our skin as well. As your largest organ, upwards of 70% of what you apply to your skin is absorbed into your body. This pertains to the products you apply directly as well as household cleaning products that come into contact with your skin on a regular basis, including laundry detergent, counter cleaners and air fresheners.

Just like real estate, it's all about location, location, location! Absorption is greatest where skin is the thinnest. From highest to lowest, this is how your body absorbs products: mucosal membranes (mouth/eyes) > genitalia/scrotum > armpits > face > back > palms/soles.

So why is this important? On a daily basis, women use an average of 12 personal care products containing 168 ingredients. Our teenage girls are using an average of 17 personal care products a day! That's a lot of products with a lot of potential absorption!

So what's the big deal? The FDA doesn't regulate the safety of ingredients in personal care products. Not to be all doom and gloom, but in the US, there are only 11 ingredients banned from use compared to the European Union which bans nearly 1,400. Crazy, right?

Why should you care? Serious and chronic illnesses have been associated with some ingredients, including cancer, neurotoxicity, immunotoxicity, hormone disruption and skin irritation. As many of these ingredients are commonly used in shampoos, body soap, deodorant, and makeup, we may unknowingly be exposing ourselves to harmful ingredients on a daily basis.

What can you do about it? Just like you would with food, read the labels of your personal care and household products. That's it. Easy peasy.

Here are 10 of the most commonly found skincare ingredients that have been identified as either causing irritation, disruption of normal bodily functioning or suspected carcinogens. The Environmental Working Group provides an excellent resource for additional information.

1. parabens (methyl, propyl, butyl, ethyl)
2. triclosan
3. peg/polyethylene glycol
4. diazolidinyl urea
5. quaternium-15
6. talc
7. imidazolindyl urea
8. toluene
9. fragrance
10. BHA/butylated hydroxyanisole

What's the silver lining? You get to choose what you put on your body. You get to choose products that maintain your skin microbiome and protective barrier and by reading all your labels, you are empowered to make safer choices. Today, there is an abundance of companies passionate about creating and curating safer products so you don't have to compromise quality or beauty by ditching your favorites. And here's the thing… You don't have to do it all at once. Start slowly. Consider the three products you use the most. Evaluate their ingredients so you can assess if you should consider an alternative.

GIVE YOURSELF AN UPGRADE

Now that you have gone through the approach, preparation, process, plan and personal care detox, it may seem like a lot to take on. I know that jumping on the bandwagon isn't always easy. Again, take it as slow or as fast as you want.

With all this information are you concerned you have to give up all the "good" stuff? Chocolate. Wine. Your favorite lipstick. I get it, believe me. But here's the thing. You don't have to give up completely the foods and products you love. Instead, give yourself an upgrade. Nearly everything you consume or use on your body or home can be made with real, simple, **whole ingredients**. Even better, purchase organic when you can find it. You deserve the best, so give yourself and your body the best you can. Starting now.

Let's say you love chocolate. I know! Rich in flavanol antioxidants, dark chocolate is good for your skin and amazing on your taste buds. You don't have to deny your love. In fact, I encourage you to embrace it, which is why I put it on your list. But give yourself an upgrade. Toss out that chocolate bar containing PGPR or TBHQ or some other alphabet soup that doesn't belong in your food. Then simply enjoy a few squares of decadent, mouth-watering organic dark chocolate from your favorite local health or whole food store. Chocolate with 70% or greater cocoa content will give you the most antioxidant bang for your buck.

Living a healthy life is not about giving up the things you love. In fact, it's exactly the opposite. Healthy living is about putting your needs, desires and happiness front and center. It means taking charge of what you can control like the food you eat, the products you use on your body and in your home, and giving them an upgrade to contain the purest, most basic, whole ingredients you can find to minimize your exposure to harmful preservatives and chemicals so you can rock on like the amazing badass you are.

Now is your time to start living your best life. The only thing you'll sacrifice are the ingredients that aren't serving your health anyway.

Ready to take action? Keep in mind that this is *your* journey and you set the pace. There is no quick fix, magic pill or potion (though topical retinoids are pretty close). Big shifts toward boosting health, vitality and happiness require taking small steps consistently. There may be missteps, side steps and complete detours and that's okay: be patient, gentle and loving towards yourself and know you are not alone. I'm here for you every step of the way.

Here are some simple, efficient and easy ways to get started today!

1. The first step is to take notice, identify and get to the foods that are hard on your gut and potentially disturbing your microbiome. Using your power of observation and jotting down your findings, you can identify patterns, triggers and exacerbating factors that will guide you moving forward.

I use a SHE sheet. A SHE sheet is nothing fancy. It's merely a simple system you too can use to move your needle towards resilient and vibrant skin and health. SHE stands for **Sleep, Hydration,** and **Eating, Emotion, Elimination.**

We will cover the importance of sleep with regards to skin health in the next chapter. For now, simply jot down the time you go to sleep and wake up daily for the next seven days. See the patterns and notice how you feel: are you energized or fatigued? Record how many ounces of water you consume daily over the course of the week. Note your skin texture, turgor and energy levels. Jot down what you are eating. Don't worry about quantity. Rather focus on how you feel after eating: satiated, elated, motivated or stuffed, bloated, anxious, and irritable. Are your bowels moving like a well-oiled machine or are you constipated feeling like you have lead bricks in your gut?

Jot it all down and remember you are merely looking for patterns, triggers and exacerbating factors so you can slowly and strategically eliminate suspected culprits of your symptoms.

2. The second step is to nourish. Below is a treasure of meals and recipes to boost your antioxidants and turn back the clock naturally. You can mix and match recipes to create a menu that will nourish you for an entire month. Use my suggestions as a guide and have fun with it.

What I've found that helps keep things simple is to assign a theme to each night of the week's meals. For example: Meatless Mondays to indulge in loads of fresh vegetables and plant-based proteins; Tacoless Tuesdays filling a bowl with gluten-free grains, protein and veggies; Wildcard Wednesdays throwing leftovers into the blender to make a soup or "garbage salad" highlighting all the tasties of the nights before; Tantalizing Thursdays to indulge your taste buds with bold flavors or a new recipe you find in a cookbook or online; Fish Fridays focusing on salmon and other fish to load up on omega-3 fatty acid. It's time to try something new! And to make it even easier to get started, go to www.drskinwhisperer.com to download your **whole foods shopping guide**. See recommendations below for some foodie website favorites.

FAVORITE FOODIE WEBSITES

Need a helping hand with where to get good info and recipes? Check out my favorites below.

https://minimalistbaker.com

https://paleoporn.com

https://www.theroastedroot.net

https://www.paleohacks.com

https://againstallgrain.com

http://tasty-yummies.com

SKIN-SAVING RECIPES

Here are some great recipes to help you get started with skin-nourishing foods. Most of these recipes, unless otherwise specified, make 3 to 4 servings depending on portion size.

Breakfasts:

Frittata

L'ego My Egg Muffins (six varieties)

Breakfast on the Fly

Green Goddess Gulp

Chocolate Decadent Delight

Lunches/Dinners:

Simple Salmon Never Tasted So Good

Turn up the Beet Bowl with Pesto and Protein

You Had Me at Curry

Just Stuff It

Mediterranean Meatballs

Flank Steak Cobbish Salad

Soups/Salads:

Super Slaw

Mason Jar Salads: Avocado Chicken Salad

Carrot Ginger Soup

Voodles

Portobello Mushroom Powerhouses

Fettuccine Bowl with Meatballs

Boosted Beverages:

Water will never be boring again!

Frittata

Ingredients:

Use any combination of veggies you have in the fridge!

- 2 tbsp organic olive, avocado or coconut oil
- 1 zucchini, chopped
- 1 green pepper, chopped
- 4 asparagus stalks
- 1/4 yellow onion, chopped
- 1 tsp kosher salt
- 1 tsp black pepper
- 4 eggs
- 2 cups fresh spinach

Instructions:

1. Preheat the oven to 375°F.
2. In a heavy skillet, add olive oil and bring to medium-low heat.
3. Sauté onions and peppers until vegetables are tender, about 7 minutes.

4. Sprinkle the mixture with salt and pepper.
5. Pour egg whites into the skillet and cook for 3 minutes.
6. Sprinkle the top with spinach.
7. Put skillet in oven and bake, uncovered, for 8 to 10 minutes. (If you use whole eggs instead of egg whites, bake at 400°F.)
8. Loosen the edges of the frittata with a rubber spatula, and then invert onto a plate.

L'ego My Egg Muffins

Makes 12 egg muffins that can be eaten for breakfast, lunch or dinner.

Ingredients:

- 12 eggs
- 1/4 tsp salt
- 1/4 tsp pepper
- 1 cup chopped cooked fish or meat (salmon, sausage, chicken, pork, steak, ground turkey)
- 1 cup diced vegetables (can be raw, sautéed or roasted, great way to use leftovers!)
- 1 handful fresh finely chopped greens (spinach, kale, collard greens, etc.)

Feel free to experiment with other herbs and spices: curry, turmeric, cumin, smoked paprika.

Instructions:

1. Preheat the oven to 350°F.
2. Grease a muffin pan with coconut oil or butter.
3. Crack eggs into large bowl and whisk with salt and pepper.
4. Divide meat, diced vegetables and chopped greens between 12 muffin cups.
5. Pour egg mixture over the veggies and meat, filling cups about 3/4 of the way.
6. Bake for approximately 20 minutes. Allow muffins to rest before using a knife to slice around the outside of the muffins and carefully removing them from the muffin tin.
7. Top with cubed avocado, hot sauce, fresh herbs or just as is. Enjoy!

Suggested veggie combinations: possibilities are endless, use your creativity and leftovers! For meats, if using sausage, bacon or deli meat remember to read labels to avoid nitrites and added sugars.

Some favorites include:

- Broccoli + mushroom + bell pepper
- Sautéed rainbow chard + asparagus + onion
- Roasted cauliflower + zucchini + spinach
- Spinach, mushroom + bell pepper
- Sautéed collard greens + celery + onion + asparagus
- Spinach + tomato + mushroom

Breakfast on the Fly

Ingredients:

- 1 avocado
- sea salt + pepper sprinkled on top

optional: dash of hot sauce or other herbs and spices

Green Goddess Gulp

Ingredients:

- 1 medium banana, previously peeled, frozen and quartered
- 1/2 cup mixed frozen berries
- 1 tbsp flaxseed meal
- 1 heaping tbsp organic salted nut butter (almond, peanut, sunflower seed)
- 1/2 to 3/4 cup unsweetened vanilla almond milk (can substitute with water, rice, hemp or coconut milk)
- 2 cups fresh spinach

optional: 1-2 tbsp protein powder* of choice

* I prefer to get protein from whole food sources but if you need an extra boost it's helpful to have some on hand. Texture and taste are often lacking with many on the market. So far, my preferred powders are Garden of Life Grain Free and Sun Warrior brands. They are organic and come in a few flavors including unflavored.

Instructions:

1. Place all ingredients in a blender (or Vitamix, Nutribullet) and blend until creamy, adding more almond milk or

frozen berries (or bananas) to thin/thicken, respectively. Serve immediately or freeze to enjoy later. As a general tip, fresh tastes best.

Other delicious combos:

- Banana + blueberry + almond butter
- Orange + mango (plus splash of lemon juice and 1 tsp fresh grated ginger)
- Pumpkin puree + banana + coconut milk (plus 1tsp pumpkin pie spice)
- Spinach + celery + cucumber + pineapple
- Kale + apple + cucumber

Chocolate Decadent Delight

Ingredients:

- 1 ripe avocado, sliced
- 1/2 large banana, peeled, sliced and frozen until hard (could use fresh and add 1/2 cup of ice)
- 2 tbsp organic cacao *or* cocoa powder
- 2 or 3 dates
- 1 cup almond milk (or other non-dairy milk)
- 1/2 tsp organic vanilla extract

Instructions

1. Place all ingredients in a blender and blend until smooth.
2. Adjust flavor/sweetness as needed.

3. Divide between two small glasses, or slurp the whole thing yourself.

Simple Salmon Never Tasted So Good

Ingredients:

- 1 to 1 and 1/2 lbs wild caught salmon (sockeye, coho, king)
- olive oil
- salt and pepper to taste

Instructions:

1. Drizzle salmon with olive oil, salt and pepper and place skin-side down on a parchment paper or foil lined baking sheet
2. Bake in the oven at 400°F for 12 to 15 minutes depending on the thickness of salmon (rule of thumb is 4 to 6 minutes for every ½ inch thickness)
3. When salmon flakes easily with a fork it's done

For **lunch** pair with asparagus, cauliflower rice or big pile of greens.

For **dinner** add on sweet potato, butternut squash, delicata squash or serve on a bed of spaghetti squash topped with pesto.

Turn Up the Beet Bowl With Basil Pesto and Protein

Ingredients

- 2 tbsp coconut oil or olive oil
- 1 small beet, peeled and chopped into quarter-inch cubes

- 1 yellow zucchini, chopped
- 2 green zucchini, chopped
- 1/4 red onion, finely chopped
- 2 to 3 cloves garlic, minced
- 1/2 head (about 4 leaves) red kale, leaves chopped
- 1 cup organic millet or organic dry short grain brown rice
- 1/3 cup basil pesto sauce store bought or homemade (recipe below) plus more for serving
- Sea salt to taste

Optional add ins: meat or fish of your preference chopped and added to bowl; or roasted pumpkin seeds

Instructions:

1. Cook the rice according to package instructions. While the rice is cooking, prepare the veggies.
2. Heat the oil over medium-high in a skillet or wok. Add the chopped beet, cover and cook, stirring occasionally, until beet turns bright red and begins to soften, about 8 minutes.
3. Add the zucchini and red onion and replace the cover. Continue cooking, stirring occasionally until the zucchini has softened but is not mushy, about 5 to 8 minutes.
4. Add the garlic and kale, cover, and cook until kale has wilted, about 2 minutes.
5. Add pesto sauce and stir together well so that everything is combined and heated through. Taste the mixture for flavor and add sea salt to taste.

6. Add in some meat or fish if desired and top with additional pesto sauce to taste.

Basil Pesto Sauce

Ingredients:

- 3 cups fresh basil leaves, packed
- 2/3 cup pine nuts
- 3 or 4 cloves garlic
- 1/4 cup olive oil (add another 1/8 to 1/4 cup if too dry)
- 1/4 tsp sea salt

Instructions:

1. Add all of the ingredients except for the oil to a food processor. Pulse 4 to 5 times to coarsely chop the ingredients.
2. After coarsely chopped, turn the food processor on and slowly pour the olive oil through the opening. Process until desired consistency is achieved.
3. Taste sauce for flavor. If desired, add additional sea salt and/or other spices.

Not in the mood for basil? No biggie. Try flat leaf parsley, cilantro, mint, sage, kale, arugula, and/or spinach as base for your pesto sauce.

No pine nuts on hand? No problem. Try raw walnuts, almonds, pecans, and/or pumpkin seeds instead.

You Had Me At Curry

Ingredients:

- 1 tbsp coconut oil
- 1 and 1/2 lbs boneless skinless chicken breast, cut into one-inch pieces
- 1 medium yellow onion, diced
- 1 green bell pepper, thinly sliced
- 1 large acorn squash, peeled, seeded, and cut into one-inch cubes (can substitute sweet potato or yam)
- 1 tsp salt
- 3 or 4 cloves garlic, minced
- one-inch piece fresh ginger, peeled and minced
- 2 to 3 tbsp Thai red curry paste (depending on preference)
- a 14-oz can full fat coconut milk (no preservatives or gums)
- 1 tbsp coconut aminos
- 2 tsp lime juice
- 1/4 cup cilantro, chopped (optional)
- handful chopped cashews (optional)
- cauliflower rice, for serving

Instructions:

1. Preheat oil in large skillet over medium heat.
2. Add chicken and cook until it's brown and completely cooked through (no pinkness).

3. Add vegetables, garlic and ginger, and cook another 2 to 3 minutes.
4. Next add the curry paste followed by the coconut milk and coconut aminos.
5. Bring to a simmer then add squash.
6. Simmer for about 20 minutes until the squash is fork-tender. Remove the pan from the heat and stir in the lime juice.
7. Taste and adjust salt and lime juice as necessary. Sprinkle with cilantro and cashews to serve.

Just Stuff It (Stuffed Peppers)

Ingredients:

- 1 lb grass-fed ground meat
- 5 large red or green bell peppers
- 1 tbsp coconut oil
- 1 medium onion, diced
- 1 cup mushrooms, chopped
- 1 cup zucchini, chopped
- 4 or 5 sprigs of asparagus, chopped
- sea salt and pepper to taste
- 1 to 2 teaspoons garlic, minced
- 1 tsp oregano
- 1 tsp dried basil (or 1 packed tbsp fresh basil then minced or chopped)

- 1 tsp smoked paprika
- 3 tbsp tomato paste (optional)

Instructions:

1. Preheat the oven to 350°F.
2. Coat a small baking dish with coconut oil.
3. Bring a large pot of water to boil. Cut the stems and very top of the peppers off, removing the seeds. Place peppers in boiling water for 4-5 minutes. Remove from the water and drain face-down on a paper towel
4. Heat the coconut oil in a large skillet over medium heat. Add onion and sauté for 3 to 4 minutes until the onion begins to soften.
5. Stir in the ground meat, oregano, basil, paprika, salt, and pepper and cook until meat is browned. Stir to break up the meat while it cooks.
6. Add the zucchini, asparagus and mushrooms to the skillet as the meat finishes cooking. Cook everything together until the vegetables are fork-tender.
7. Remove the pan from heat and drain any juices from the pan. Once drained, this is where you would add tomato paste, if desired.
8. Ready for assembly: place the peppers upright in the baking dish and spoon the meat mixture into the center of each.
9. Bake for 15 minutes.

Mediterranean Meatballs

These meatballs are amazing on their own or layered on a bed of spaghetti squash, zucchini noodles, on salads, in soups or with eggs for breakfast. Makes 12 to 14 meatballs depending on size.

Ingredients:

- 1 lb grass fed ground meat (beef, lamb, turkey, chicken)
- 1/2 medium white onion, minced
- 1 and 1/2 tsp dried oregano
- 1 tsp sea salt
- 1 tsp ground black pepper
- 1 tsp dried thyme
- 1 and 1/2 tbsp smoked paprika powder
- 1/4 tsp ground cinnamon
- 1/4 tsp ground nutmeg
- 1/4 cup chopped fresh parsley

Instructions:

1. Add all ingredients together in a bowl and mix well to combine. Evenly divide mixture into half-inch to one-inch meatballs.
2. Heat outdoor grill or grill pan on stove top to medium-high heat.
3. Cook meatballs for 2 to 3 minutes on each side for medium doneness or until cooked to preference.
4. Serve with toppings and dipping sauce of choice (see condiment page).

Flank Steak Cobbish Salad

Ingredients:

- 1 to 1 and 1/2 lbs grass-fed flank steak
- 1/2 cup olive oil
- 3 cloves garlic, minced
- 1 tsp salt
- 1 tsp black pepper
- 1/2 cup onion, chopped
- 1/3 cup red or white wine vinegar
- 4 hard-boiled eggs, halved or quartered
- 1 cup cherry tomatoes, halved
- 1/2 cup red onion, chopped
- 8 cups romaine lettuce or mixed greens, chopped
- 2 medium avocados, sliced or chopped

Instructions:

Combine first seven ingredients in a Pyrex dish and let marinate at least 4 hours or overnight.

1. Remove steak from marinade and grill to desired doneness.
2. Let rest and slice into strips.
3. Per serving, put 2 cups of the lettuce into a bowl. Top with tomatoes, onion, egg, avocado and steak, arranging as desired.
4. Serve with your favorite dressing

Amp up the salad with a serving of baked or roasted sweet potato, cubed butternut squash, delicata squash.

Salads, Soups & Veggie Sides

Any of these recipes can be used for lunch, dinner or a side. For main lunch and dinner meals, add a protein source. You can also round out the meal with a carb (sweet potato, gluten-free grain: millet, rice, amaranth, quinoa) and you are set!

Super Slaw

Ingredients:

- 3 to 4 cups of kale, washed, stems removed (approx 1 bunch)
- 2 cups red cabbage, washed
- 2 cups green cabbage, washed
- 1 medium head of broccoli (approx 2-3 cups), washed
- 4 cloves roasted garlic (depending on preference, can add more, whole head is 12 cloves)
- 1/3 cup olive oil
- 1/3 cup apple cider or white balsamic vinegar
- juice of 1/2 lemon
- 2 tbsp fresh rosemary, washed
- smoked paprika and cumin to taste

optional: a quarter-cup raw pepitas (pumpkin seeds)

Instructions:

1. Put all veggies in a large food processor and pulse until shredded.
2. Transfer veggies to a large mixing bowl.
3. For the dressing, add garlic cloves, oil, vinegar, lemon juice, rosemary and any other spices to a blender and pulse until rosemary is pulverized.
4. To serve, pour dressing into bowl with veggies and mix until well combined.
5. Sprinkle pumpkin seeds on top of individual servings.

Portobello Mushroom Powerhouses

Ingredients:

- 4 Portobello mushrooms, stems removed
- 2 tbsp melted ghee, butter, coconut or olive oil
- sea salt and pepper to taste
- 1 tsp dried herbs (thyme, rosemary, basil)

Toppings: get creative and enjoy!

Below are a few favorite combos:

- Spinach + cooked butternut squash + caramelized onions
- Sautéed rainbow chard + asparagus + onion
- Pesto + chicken + roasted red peppers
- Sautéed kale + cooked sweet potato + zucchini

Instructions:

1. Preheat oven to 350°F and line a baking sheet with parchment paper.
2. Remove stems of the mushrooms and scrape out the "gills" with a spoon. Rub each mushroom top and side with olive or coconut oil. Place gill side down and use a knife to make a shallow X on top of each mushroom. Season with salt and pepper to taste and dried herbs, if desired.
3. Once seasoned, place mushrooms gill side up and roast for 10-15 minutes to allow for juices to evaporate.
4. After 10-15 minutes, flip mushrooms so they are gill side down and continue roasting for 10 more minutes.
5. While mushroom are cooking prepare other toppings or raid fridge for leftovers you can reheat to add on top when mushrooms are done.
6. Once mushrooms are finished cooking, pile on the toppings to build your slider.
7. If you are adding a sauce or need to reheat a condiment, place slider back in oven for 3 to 5 minutes until sauce or condiment heats up. Pair with a bed of greens or other veggies and enjoy!

Mason Jar Salads

Possibilities are endless with these mason jar salads. Mix and match veggies, protein and dressings for lunch at work or at home. Avocado chicken spinach below is just one example. Check out Pinterest for tons of ideas.

Avocado Chicken Spinach Salad

Ingredients:

For two jars of salad:

- 1/2 cup cucumber
- 1/2 cup celery, sliced
- 1/2 cup bell pepper, chopped
- 1/2 cup cherry tomatoes
- 2 tbsp black or Kalamata olives
- 1/2 cup chopped chicken

For the avocado spinach dressing:

- 1/2 cup fresh packed spinach
- 1/2 ripe avocado
- juice of 1 lemon
- 2 tbsp extra virgin olive oil
- 1/2 tsp salt
- 1/4 tsp pepper

Instructions:
1. Spiral, shred or thinly slice zucchini. Set aside.
2. Add dressing ingredients to food processor or high speed blender and mix until smooth.
3. Pour half the dressing into the bottom of two mason jars.
4. Add celery on top of dressing.

5. Add peppers on top of celery then top with chicken.
6. Add tomatoes and olives.
7. Lastly, add half the spiraled zucchini into each mason jar.
8. Cover and refrigerate. Lasts up to 5 days.
9. Once ready to eat, shake the jar vigorously then pour onto a plate. Toss with fork if needed to mix dressing.

Carrot Ginger Soup

Ingredients:

- 2 tbsp coconut oil
- 1 medium red onion
- 3 cloves garlic, minced
- 3 tbsp ginger, minced
- 2 lbs carrots, peeled and chopped
- 4 cups vegetable or chicken broth
- 1 tsp cinnamon
- 1 tsp salt
- 4 tbsp chives or dill, finely chopped (for garnish)

Instructions:

1. Heat oil over medium-high heat in a large pot.
2. Add the onions and cook for 1 to 2 minutes.
3. Stir in the ginger and garlic, and cook for another 1 to 2 minutes.

4. Add the carrots and cook another 10 minutes, stirring often.

5. Next add the broth, cinnamon and salt and bring the pot to a boil. Once boiling, turn down to low simmer, cover pot and cook for additional 20 to 30 minutes, until the carrots have completely softened.

6. At this point, remove pot from heat and blend the soup with an immersion blender or transfer to a high-powered blender. Blend the soup until it's pureed to your desired consistency.

7. Serve with garnish.

For a twist on flavor, try roasting veggies first, then add seasoning and broth to high speed blender. Or how about serving with side of meatballs, chicken and greens?

"Voodles": Veggie Alternative to Pasta Noodles

Suggestions of veggies to make voodles:

- zucchini or yellow squash
- sweet potato or yam
- cucumber
- daikon radish
- beets

Instructions:

1. Use a spiralizer attachment for food processor, a handheld spiralizer tool or your basic veggie peeler (to create veggie ribbons).

2. Serve raw or sauté and pile on your toppings.

Check out this post for additional recipes and ideas: http:/blog.paleohacks.com/noodle-recipes

"Fettucine" Bowls with Meatballs

Ingredients for two large servings:

- 4 yellow squash
- 1 zucchini, 1 bell pepper, 1 eggplant (or other assorted veggies), chopped into bite-sized pieces
- 1 cup tomato sauce (no added sugar)
- Mediterranean meatballs
- sea salt and pepper to taste
- 1 to 2 tbsp olive oil

Instructions:

1. Preheat oven to 350°F and line a baking sheet with parchment paper.
2. Toss veggies in a bowl and drizzle with olive oil, salt and pepper. Stir to ensure veggies are coated with oil and seasoning.
3. Transfer veggies to baking sheet and roast for 35 minutes or until done to preference.

Boosted Beverages

Add some flavor to your cold beverages easily with flavored ice cubes. Combine filtered water with sliced, chopped or pureed fruits and herbs, fill your ice cube trays and boom! You have a boosted beverage. Enjoy!

Have fun with this and try all sorts of combinations. Below are a few suggestions to get you started:

- Cucumber and mint
- Orange and ginger
- Orange and rosemary
- Strawberry and basil
- Lime and basil
- Kiwi and pineapple
- Blueberry and mint

Bon appétit!

Chapter 5:
BEAUTY SLEEP IS REAL

"Sleep is the golden chain that ties health and our bodies together."

Thomas Dekker

Tossing and turning was the norm, the snooze button habitual, followed by reluctantly dragging myself out of bed when the alarm went off again and again. Staring back at me in the mirror were puffy eyes sitting on top of dark circles cradled by fine lines etched into the skin. Staying up late from either being on hospital call or trying to cram in my studies to be prepared for the next day's rounds put me on a constant rollercoaster of late nights, early mornings and poor sleep quality. I would like to stay this ended when I completed my residency, but habits are hard to break. I stayed on this train for more than a decade after I finished my training. Despite having the knowledge of how important sleep is for our overall health and our skin, it took being diagnosed with skin cancer to knock me over the head with a reminder that I needed to get off the ride I was on.

The whole of life is guided by a rhythm. The ocean ebbs and flows with rising and receding water levels washing ashore. We call them tides, but they are a reflection of how our lives are designed too. Put in context, this is the way we alternate between periods of sleep and wakefulness, the rhythm closely linked to the occurrence of day and night. If you have ever traveled and experienced jet lag, you are intimately familiar with the effects of disturbing these rhythms. By altering sleep, jet lag impacts your ability to think clearly and effectively, affects your mood and interpersonal relationships, and causes a drop in the general quality of your life. Thankfully, after a few days, we recover and get back on track, but imagine if this were to last for weeks, months or years on end? Our lives would be completely disrupted. I, for one, can relate. And this is the unfortunate reality for approximately 60% of adults who experience sleep problems at least several nights a week. Are you one of them?

Our body has a pattern, called the circadian rhythm, which is controlled by a master clock in the hypothalamus part of your brain called the suprachiasmatic nucleus (SCN). The SCN is located just behind your eyes. As light filters in from the eyes, the SCN initiates signals to other parts of your brain, setting off a regulated pattern of activities that affect your entire body. Once exposed to the first light each day, your circadian clock begins performing functions like raising your body temperature and releasing hormones. Two of the most important hormones that impact your sleep are cortisol and melatonin. Cortisol, made by your adrenal glands, synchronizes many of the clocks in other parts of the body, and helps regulate your blood sugar and levels of stress and inflammation. Melatonin is produced by various tissues in the body, including your skin, although the major source is the pineal gland of your brain. The production and release of melatonin from the pineal gland occurs with a distinct daily rhythm, peak levels occurring at night. It has numerous functions including influencing your body weight, reproduction, anti-jet lag effects and hair growth, and helping your body know when to sleep and wake up.

Besides adjusting the timing of your master clock, bright light has another effect. It directly inhibits the release of melatonin. This is important, because melatonin is only produced in the dark. Even if the pineal gland is "switched on" by the clock, it will not produce melatonin unless your environment is dark enough. Both sunlight and artificial lighting from overhead and digital sources can prevent the release of melatonin.

So when things get in the way — jet lag, staying up late to watch your favorite show, surfing the internet into the wee hours, or worrying about a work deadline — you can disrupt your circadian rhythm.

Why does this matter? Because disrupted circadian rhythms may contribute to a variety of adverse health effects including obesity, diabetes, cardiovascular disease, depression and Alzheimer's disease. Sleep impacts your life, health and wellbeing in ways you may appreciate, but there are other impacts you should know, especially as they pertain to your skin health. Let's explore them all.

WHAT HAPPENS WHEN YOU DON'T GET ENOUGH SLEEP?

Sleep is vital to your overall health and wellbeing, because it's a time for rest and repair. When you don't get enough, your ability to function quickly deteriorates and eventually crumbles. High quality restful sleep enables you not only to survive, but to thrive. Sleep is the time your body heals damaged cells, recovers from the day's activities, and recharges your body for the next day. It enhances your productivity and performance, and ignites your creativity.

Sleep restores your body and your mind, rejuvenating your physical function while amplifying your mental and emotional fortitude. It protects against illness, supports your bone and heart health and boosts your immune system and metabolism. Sleep keeps your skin looking young and helps protect you from various forms of cancer, including breast, ovarian, uterine, colon and skin cancer. Bottom line: virtually every bodily function, emotion and relationship you have is affected by sleep.

In addition to feeling drowsy, having brain fog and your mood being off-track, a lack sleep can have a significant impact on skin function and aging.

A lack of sleep disrupts your usual daily hormone patterns causing cortisol to increase and melatonin to decrease. The result is heightened stress and inflammation in your body. For your skin, this can manifest as a worsening of inflammatory skin conditions, including acne, eczema and psoriasis. And it's not just a one-way mechanism. An exacerbation of eczema, for example, can lead to increased itching, which can further disrupt sleep. A vicious cycle begins.

With sleep's important role in boosting immunity, its deficiency can make your skin more vulnerable to infection, irritation and exacerbate skin conditions that have an underlying autoimmunity issue going on, such as psoriasis.

During sleep, your skin rebalances its hydration status and increases its capacity to retain water to keep your skin supple and moisturized. A lack of sleep interferes with proper water balance resulting in puffiness, dryness and visible wrinkles.

Sleep plays a key role in rejuvenating your skin due to the interaction of melatonin with the cells in your epidermis and dermis. Melatonin protects your epidermal cells against cell death, while stimulating the growth of your fibroblasts. Fibroblasts are responsible for production of your collagen and elastin, which you might recall from earlier are the keys to firm, supple and youthful skin.

Sleep is also the time when growth hormone, which plays a central role in cell repair, is at its peak. Without sufficient sleep, your skin's ability to rejuvenate and repair damage is compromised. Studies have shown that a deficiency in melatonin reduces skin thickness, delays wound healing, and induces skin degenerative changes. Fine lines, uneven pigmentation, decreased elasticity, scar formation and wrinkles are the result.

One of the most important roles that melatonin plays in your skin's health is its ability to help protect it from environmental stressors, especially UV radiation. The fact that your skin can receive melatonin from your circulation as well as be a source of production highlights the significant role melatonin plays in regulating your skin's structure and function. As such, it's considered one of your body's most potent antioxidants. In fact, melatonin has been shown to be a stronger scavenger of free radicals than vitamin C or vitamin E, both of which have been used to treat cell damage.

Melatonin is a highly lipophilic hormone, which means it can easily cross the cellular membranes and protect your vital intracellular structures including your DNA and your mitochondria, which are your cells' energy powerhouses. As an antioxidant, melatonin has a protective role against UVB skin damage and can lessen that oxidative stress mentioned earlier. It exerts its antioxidant effects by blocking free radical damage, decreasing inflammation and stimulating the formation of other potent antioxidants in the body, like glutathione and superoxide dismutase. In turn, these antioxidants provide even more support in blocking the damaging effects of UV rays. In fact, studies show that pre-treating skin with topical melatonin strongly protects it against sunburn.

Even more exciting is current research on topical melatonin and oral melatonin supplementation to prevent and treat skin cancer.

In addition to all of the skin benefits that sleep can provide to help you look younger and stay safe in the sun, it's worth mentioning that sleep also is good for your waistline, which keeps you looking younger and feeling healthier too. When you don't get enough sleep and your cortisol and insulin levels increase, it prompts your body to store energy as fat, especially in your abdomen. Sleep also regulates the hormones that control your hunger and feelings of fullness. Ghrelin, the hormone that stimulates hunger, increases. Simultaneously, leptin, the hormone that promotes a feeling of fullness, decreases. On top of this, as cortisol increases, it triggers a need for serotonin, which is a brain chemical that influences your mood and hunger; this may well be the reason you crave carbs and fat when you are tired.

Based on the current sleep research, the average ideal amount of time you should be sleeping is between 7 and 9 hours. As with most everything, it is just as much about quality as it is quantity, so how can I help you achieve both? Below is what I have found to be the most efficient, most effective ways to get deep restful sleep consistently.

HOW TO IMPROVE YOUR SLEEP

Creating an environment that appeals to all your senses is the easiest way to promote good sleep and get your restful zzzs.

Sight

As light is the single most important factor regulating your circadian rhythm and release of melatonin, filtering out light that could impact your ability to get a good night's rest is top priority.

Blue light emitted from digital devices like your cell phone and computer have been found to suppress melatonin production twice as much as other wavelengths of light, so it's important to decrease your exposure when preparing for sleep. Easy ways you can do this include: adding filters to your phone and computers using apps like f.lux and software such as Apple's Night shift; wearing glasses that block blue light wavelengths in the evening; eating foods rich in the carotenoids lutein and zeaxanthin that can protect your eyes and boost their natural ability to block out blue light; making your bedroom as dark as possible by using blackout curtains or wearing an eye mask. You can also minimize overhead lighting by using a Himalayan salt lamp at your bedside to provide a warm amber glow to usher you into a slumber.

Sound

Some sounds can be soothing while others can be disruptive to your sleep, so blocking out the disruptive ones with ear plugs or a white noise machine may help.

Touch

Being comfortable in bed is crucial to ensuring a good night's rest. Choosing sheets, pillows and a mattress that ooze comfort will make a big difference. As will extremes in temperature, which is why keeping your room between 65°F to 75°F is optimal. Personally, I love to use a device called a Chilipad to help me regulate my bed temperature.

Getting some good loving reduces stress and releases the feel-good hormone oxytocin, so don't overlook the benefit of a good romp before sleep time.

Smell

Your sense of smell is one of your most powerful. Just like sound, certain smells can work for you or against you as you try to drift off to sleep. Consider opening your window or getting an air filter, not only to improve the quality of your air, but also to filter out any unwanted odors. The use of aromatherapy either with a diffuser or applied topically can also create a soothing environment with lavender being notorious for aiding rest, relaxation and sleep.

Taste

Eating too close to your bedtime or overstuffing your belly can make sleep more challenging. The same goes for consumption of caffeine and alcohol. While I am a big fan of the skin cancer preventative benefits of coffee and the resveratrol in red wine, they create challenges for getting restful sleep when consumed too close to bedtime. With caffeine's half-life of 8 to 10 hours, it is best to have your last cup no later 2pm and your last alcoholic beverage 3 hours before your plan to go to bed.

Personally, one of the most impactful changes I have made to improve my sleep quality is increasing my consumption of magnesium. Magnesium is considered an essential mineral, meaning we have to get it from outside sources as our body cannot produce it. Having a role in over 300 different functions in the body, including stabilizing moods, keeping stress levels in check and aiding sleep, low levels of magnesium can throw our bodies out of whack. Magnesium supports restful sleep by maintaining levels of a brain chemical called GABA, which promotes relaxation, reduces stress and assists sleep.

Magnesium-rich foods include:

- dark leafy greens (kale)
- nuts and seeds (almond, cashew, sunflower and sesame)
- squash
- broccoli
- meat
- chocolate
- coffee

Oral supplementation of magnesium is an option as well, with a general guideline of 100 to 350 mg daily but individual dosing will vary depending on an individual's magnesium level. As with all vitamins and supplements you should check in with your physician to make sure it is appropriate for your situation. There are certain conditions that are associated with higher risks for magnesium deficiency, like diabetes and alcoholism, as well as conditions that reduce the amount of magnesium the body absorbs, like inflammatory bowel disease and stomach infections. Add to this medications that can interact with magnesium like antibiotics and certain blood pressure medications and you can see why it's important to make sure supplementation is safe for you to begin.

Ready to get better sleep?

Here is your checklist for sleeping and waking better:

1. Have a consistent sleep and wake schedule even on weekends. You can use the "bedtime" setting on your smart phone clock to help you with this.

2. Get sun exposure in the morning... get the benefit without the burn.
3. Watch the sunrise and the sunset whenever possible.
4. Limit screen time 2 hours before bed.
5. To automatically regulate blue light being emitted from your computer screen, download this application: www.justgetflux.com.
6. Turn on "Night Shift" if you have an iPhone or download "Twilight" for your Android phone. These apps will regulate the light coming from your screen automatically based on the time of day.
7. Limit your EMF (electro-magnetic field) exposure. Put your phone in airplane mode and charge devices outside of bedroom.
8. Wind down your day by winding down your overhead lighting. Reduce or eliminate overhead lighting in the evenings to help your brain acclimate to night time. Create a soothing environment with candlelight, use a salt lamp or wear blue-light blocking glasses.
9. Before getting into bed, sit down and spill out all your worries, to-do lists, ruminations and big dreams into a journal. Let the pages be the receptacle for the vortex of thoughts running through your mind so when you get into bed you can truly relax, rest and repair knowing you having already addressed your thoughts.
10. Based on your observations from your SHE sheet in Chapter 4, if you are not banking 7 to 9 hours of quality sleep, dial in your bedtime to 15 minutes earlier each night until you reach a sweet spot in this range.

11. Use your bedroom for sleep and good lovin' only. Get rid of your TV.
12. Use a Himalayan salt lamp in the morning and evening to gently wake you at the beginning of the day and put you to bed at night.

Sweets dreams!

Chapter 6:
STRESS PERCEPTION

"Miracles happen every day. Change your perception of what a miracle is and you'll see them all around you."

Jon Bon Jovi

Have you ever frantically rushed around your house looking for your keys or glasses, only to find they have been in your pocket or on top of your head the entire time? In anticipatory excitement of a big event, you look in the mirror and discover that you have broken out with the biggest pimple you have ever seen, your eczema has flared up or you have broken out in hives? This is the impact of stress.

As dermatologists, Drs. Stokes and Pillsbury noted back in the 1930s, there is an intimate relationship between our gut, brain and skin. Not only is stress a major cause of sleep problems, it is responsible for upwards of 90% of all doctors' visits, emphasizing the significant role that our thoughts, diets and environments can play in our overall health, wellbeing and the appearance of our skin.

Remember, when you experience stress, whether real or perceived, your sympathetic nervous system switches on. Your body prepares itself for attack. Dating back to prehistoric times, that attack was likely to be by something like a saber-toothed tiger; in order to survive, you would have had to either fight it, flee as fast as you could or freeze where you were. Fast forward to the modern day and though that tiger may not be chasing you, your response to a perceived threat remains the same. When you are in this mode, your body has a specific series of actions it takes towards regulating your mood, motivation and fear to ensure your survival. We discussed what happens to your digestion in these moments back in Chapter 4, but how does stress and the resulting hormone release affect other aspects of your body's function?

When stress levels soar, your hypothalamus, a tiny region at the base of your brain, sounds off an alarm system in your body. This triggers a series of events in your nerve and hormone signaling, which prompts your adrenal glands, located on top of your kidneys, to release a surge of hormones including cortisol and adrenaline. Adrenaline increases your heart rate, elevates your blood pressure and amps up your energy supplies. Cortisol, your primary stress hormone, increases sugar in the bloodstream and creates imbalances in your other hormones including progesterone, testosterone and thyroid, leading to suppression of the reproductive and growth processes. Increased cortisol levels also alter your immune system responses producing increased levels of inflammation. Chronic inflammation has been discovered to be the root cause of many diseases, including heart disease, autoimmune disorders and cancer. It is also thought to be at the core of skin aging, including sagging skin, wrinkles, discoloration, enlarged pores and lack of that radiant glow. The vicious cycle of chronic inflammation exacerbates skin conditions including acne, psoriasis and atopic dermatitis, and interferes with wound healing. So to recap: stress can wreak havoc on your body, mind and skin.

In our daily lives, rushing around from one thing to next, we feel constantly bombarded by stressors that cause a physical, mental or emotional response. Now, stress is a natural part of life and not something we can avoid completely, nor should we. Stress can serve as a motivator to implement change, make big shifts in your business and personal life, and it can set you on a new course you never thought possible. That said, in our current culture, there has been emphasis on reducing, managing or ridding ourselves of stress in order to achieve health and wellness. When you are just trying to get through your day and feel like you are getting pummeled by stressors from every direction, the pressure to reduce stress may actually cause more stress. And who needs that?

Let's explore why we feel emotional stress. Most of the time we experience the sensation of being stressed because we are unsure what the outcome of a situation might be. We are lacking clarity on how we should approach a situation or how we are going to resolve it. We look towards our past for evidence on how situations played out and use those past outcomes to determine our present and predict the future, even if they are irrelevant to the situation at hand. We tend to get overwhelmed by the how, and as a result, we experience a feeling of being stuck and struggling.

Let's look at a hypothetical example of how this plays out. You are down to the wire on a deadline at work and still have a lot to get done to complete the job. Your mind starts racing to the what-ifs... *What if I can't meet the deadline? If I can't meet the deadline, my boss will be mad at me. What if my boss is mad at me and pulls me from the project? If she pulls me from the project, I'll lose the client. If I lose the client, how will I make enough money to cover my expenses?* You can imagine that there is a never-ending rabbit hole of questions you could create in that scenario. But here's the thing.

The only part of this equation that is true in this scenario is that there is a deadline that needs to be met. All of what followed was a fabrication of the mind; what *could* happen if the objective measure was not met. The line of questioning created the lens through which the experience was interpreted: one of anxiety, overwhelm and stagnation. In other words, it created a **sensation of stress**.

But what if you approached it from another angle? What if the perceived obstacle of a deadline wasn't actually an obstacle, rather an opportunity to ask a different set of questions? If it's possible to ask questions that can stop you in your tracks and create a total sense of overwhelm, would you entertain the possibility that asking different questions could produce a different outcome? A helpful outcome.

Let's take a look at that scenario again and change the questions being asked. What if you completed the project and your boss was ecstatic with the work you produced? How would that impact your life? It could provide a sense of joy, accomplishment, and certainty that you could secure the client and have the resources to pay your expenses. So what do you need to do to make this happen? What steps would you need to take? You would start asking yourself totally different questions, right? Here are some examples. *How would I need to prioritize the tasks in the project to ensure they get completed? How would I delegate my time to address those tasks? What is the first step I need to take to put this plan in motion?*

Rather than asking questions through a negative lens, together we have just generated an empowering line of questioning that pointed to a subsequent series of action steps to address the situation. Asking empowering questions changes the perception of the experience. The obstacle is no longer an obstacle. Rather than serving as a source of stress, taking a different approach provided an **opportunity to gain clarity**.

Can you think of a scenario in your life where you could apply this technique? In the space below, jot down one thing that has had you riled up, spinning your wheels or pulling out your hair in the last few weeks, days or hours. We will call this your trigger.

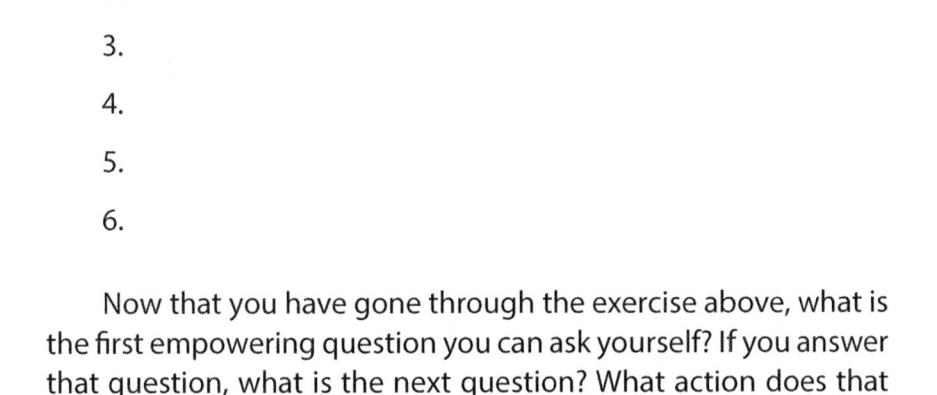

Trigger:

1.

2.

3.

4.

5.

6.

Now that you have gone through the exercise above, what is the first empowering question you can ask yourself? If you answer that question, what is the next question? What action does that answer lead you towards? What happens next? In the space below, make note of the empowering questions you have come up with and the action steps that arose from your questions.

Empowering questions:

1.

2.

3.

4.

5.

6.

Trigger:

1.

2.

3.

4.

5.

6.

Using this technique will enable you to switch out of your fight, flee or freeze state and switch into your relaxation state knowing you are capable of generating a *plan of action*. Questions can help bring clarity to a situation. All it takes is the right line of questioning. Questions allow you to acknowledge where you are in your thought process as well as help you define where you want to go to achieve your desired outcome.

While we cannot avoid stress in our lives, we can change how we perceive it and the meaning we give to any experience. By going through the exercise of the two hypothetical scenarios and your own real one, you can now appreciate that stress does not have to be a source of paralysis. Rather it can be a catalyst for action.

In every aspect of your life, you have the power to generate questions that can propel you forward to achieve whatever goal you set for yourself. This is the path toward creating the life you crave and truly living it. It is also the underpinning for keeping you and your skin healthy, radiant and looking younger.

Swift Skin Action
Download your free worksheets and come up with your own plan of action!

www.drskinwhisperer.com

Chapter 7:
ART OF COMMUNICATION

"The most important thing in communication is hearing what isn't said."

Peter Drucker

Your body is in a constant state of replacing itself. Your cells communicate with each other and their environment to get important information. Based on the information they receive, they carry out specific functions, ranging from repair and survival to programmed cell death. Did you know that signals communicating your positive and negative thoughts influence cell function? This is a profound notion that your body can change as you retrain your thinking.

Hectic schedules, social obligations, financial pressures, kids' activities… It's understandable that many people live in a constant state of sending distress signals to their body. But here's the thing, we know that healing cannot take place in this state. The ability to heal flourishes when we send signals that facilitate our body's ability to rest, digest and repair. To heal, we need to switch on our parasympathetic state.

Positive communication is the key to healthy relationships, especially the relationship between you and your body, your body and its cellular constituents, your body and your mind.

You have already begun your journey of improving the communication between you and your body and your cells by taking notice of the facets of your life. Trust in your body should be greater now you're taking notice of what your skin is revealing about what your body needs in the form of nutrient-dense foods, sleep of sufficient quantity and quality, and reframing your stressors. Now let us begin the journey of exploring your communication between your body and your mind.

To better understand your means of communication with yourself, first it is important to take notice of how you communicate with other people. This may seem counterintuitive but indulge me for a moment, because I believe that how you communicate with others is a reflection of how you communicate with yourself. First, take a moment to reflect on the people with whom you spend your time and who you are when you're with them. Think about the three to five people with whom you spend the most time. Notice how you feel and behave in your skin. Do you like how you feel? Do you feel authentic, elated, supported and creative or do you feel deflated, dejected, angry or resentful? Acknowledge and celebrate yourself for being honest and raising your awareness.

Feeling comfortable with who you are is critical to creating the life you crave. To live into it, you need to believe you deserve it and that it is within your reach.

As I shared in the introduction, for much of my young life, I didn't feel comfortable in my skin because I was teased for what was on it. I used my interpretation of my experience to craft my story that if what was on my skin was displeasing to others, then I as a person must also be displeasing to them. As a result, I became a person whose mission it was to "please." I became a diligent rule-follower, an excellent student, a dutiful assistant and a trusted confidante. I changed who I was being with others to reinforce the story I had created. The problem was that it didn't make me feel any better about myself. In fact, it made me feel worse on many levels. Sure, being a "pleaser" helped me achieve good grades and kept me out of trouble, but my self-esteem and confidence still suffered. The person I was *being* was not the person I was meant to be; it was who I thought I *should* be.

No one is immune to emotional scars or traumas. We have all had experiences that have made an impact on our lives whether in childhood or as adults. It's how we've chosen to interpret those experiences that guides our choices from that point forward. Similar to what I discussed with how we perceive stress, so too how we think, feel and act are all tied to our interpretation of an experience, which then determines the outcome.

WHAT ARE LIMITING BELIEFS?

You may already be familiar with the concept of **limiting beliefs**. If not, allow me to take a moment to review this important and powerful idea as it is the cornerstone to our self-esteem, self-image and ability not only to create the life we crave but to live it too. Limiting beliefs are simply the stories we tell ourselves that hold us back from being successful in life. Being successful is not defined as having prestige, power and money, though these may be by-products. Being successful is living your life in alignment with your passions, your purpose and your authentic unapologetically sexy self — confident and comfortable in who you are in your skin.

Each of us has created an image of ourselves and the type of person "we are." This image has been created from our own beliefs about ourselves. But here's the thing that is so vital to understand: Most of these beliefs about ourselves have been unconsciously formed from our past experiences. They have been generated from our humiliations, our successes, our failures, our glory and the way other people have reacted to us, especially in early childhood. It is from these experiences that we construct our self-image and we believe that it represents the **truth of who we are**. This image becomes the axis around which our entire personality, behavior and circumstances revolve.

In other words, your beliefs about who you are determine the thoughts you have about yourself, which in turn fuel your emotions, which dictates your behavior and governs your outcomes. Each outcome you achieve serves to reinforce your belief. Depending on the image you have created about yourself, this can create either a vicious or benevolent cycle. You see, your brain is a goal-achieving machine that can either work *for* you as a success machine or *against* you as a failure machine, depending on how you operate it and the goals you set for it. Your brain will seek and use evidence from your past to support the goal you set to create your outcome.

For example, a common limiting belief is one of not feeling "good enough." Hypothetically speaking, let's say you are in the running for a job promotion, but the running dialogue in your head is that you are not qualified for the position and don't have the experience to succeed at it. You show up to the interview lacking the confidence and conviction that you deserve the job. When you find out you got passed over for the promotion, it reinforces your belief that you were not "good enough" to get it. Or perhaps as someone who sees herself as the sort of person nobody likes, your friend finds people avoid her at the networking event she attends. This objective "proof" reinforces the image she has of herself as "unlikeable."

Here's the amazing thing about all of this, just as you create your self-image from your past experiences, you can change it by the same process. However, until you take notice of your own limiting beliefs, you cannot fully appreciate how much they could be holding you back from being successful, nor can you change them.

Below are a few commonly held limiting beliefs. Do any of them resonate with you?

1. Things never work out for me.
2. I don't know how to do it and I'll do it wrong.
3. I'm not [smart, good looking, strong, slender, talented ...] enough.
4. Other people can accomplish that but I can't.
5. There is nothing I can do about my [marriage, health, career, finances…].
6. I can't trust anyone.

What other beliefs do you hear yourself saying and believe to be true? Write them below:

1.
2.
3.
4.
5.
6.

This may not be an exhaustive list and I recommend that you continue to take notice of beliefs that may come up in your day-to-day activities over time. I encourage you to do this without judging or berating yourself. Rather, use it as an opportunity to simply become aware of your beliefs so you can address them.

Now that you have identified some of your beliefs, which you have held to be true up until this point, I am going to ask you to shift gears and make a new type of list. This time you are tapping into another aspect of the gut-brain connection, your intuition, AKA "your gut."

Without thinking and without analyzing, complete the sentences below. Just write the first thing that crosses your mind:

1. My gut tells me:

2. My gut tells me:

3. My gut tells me:

4. My gut tells me:

5. My gut tells me:

6. My gut tells me:

Now, take your list of limiting beliefs and compare them to your gut instincts. What do you see? Is there a discrepancy between what you believe to be true and what your intuition is telling you? Based on my experience, doing this work with clients and completing this exercise myself, there is usually a huge disconnect between the two. The beliefs typically reflect a negative perception of self, while the gut instinct responses are nurturing and positive.

This is what I want you to know: your intuition or gut instinct is your truth, not your limiting beliefs. Tapping into your intuition is tapping into your wisdom and it is what your true self has been saying all along, but you haven't been open to receiving it. It is the whisper you couldn't hear, but now, in this moment, it is shouting to get your attention. This is the new foundation upon which you can build your self-image, boost your self-esteem, and acknowledge yourself for being the amazing and dynamic creator you are. It is from this space that you can generate positive thoughts to fuel loving emotion, which can drive massive action to produce powerful results.

CREATE THE LIFE YOU CRAVE

To create the life you crave, you have to have clarity about what you want your life to look like. Most of us, until we recognize that we have limiting beliefs, don't fully appreciate the ways in which they are holding us back. To clarify what you want for yourself in the present and future, take notice of where you are right now in your life so you can decide where you want to be. I call this "crave creation."

Below, I invite you to rank each facet of your current life from 1 to 10 and in the next column repeat your ranking for what you want each to be. In other words, ***create your crave***. The designation "1" means this area needs a major upgrade and "10" is total bliss. Some areas of your life may already be a 10. Acknowledge and celebrate this! For areas that are not at your ideal number, there's an opportunity to work towards bringing them into balance with the rest.

Your NOW	Your CRAVE
Family	Family
Professional	Professional
Health	Health
Spiritual	Spiritual
Financial	Financial
Social	Social
Relationships	Relationships
Charitable contribution	Charitable contribution
Love	Love

How does it feel to have a clearer picture of the areas in your life where you want an upgrade? Remember, when you take notice, you can take action.

If you are willing to concede that your beliefs aren't the truth and your intuition is, you open the door to creating anything you can imagine, including your upgrades. Remember, your brain is a goal-achieving machine. It searches your past for evidence to support the goals you set for yourself. Can you think of an experience where you had success and felt good about yourself? No accomplishment is too small. Did you learn how to ride a bike, drive a car, figure out how to spell your name? All you need is one positive experience, regardless of how long ago it occurred, to remind you that you can accomplish your goals. You don't need an experience that parallels what you are trying to create right now, just a reminder of how you felt when you achieved that goal to create a positive shift in your self-image.

Now, here's the best news! Not only is your brain a goal-achieving machine, but also studies have shown that it can't tell the difference between images that are real or imagined. This means it doesn't matter if what you crave for your life doesn't even exist yet. You can create it and live into it. The most powerful way to create is through visualization. I will walk you through a visualization exercise below so you can begin creating.

To give you a better sense of what I'm proposing, let's visualize improving your health with increased energy, elevated mood and a revving libido as an example of the process.

Take a delicious deep breath in through your nose and out through your mouth. Inhale for a count of 4 and exhale for a count of 6. Inhale for a count of 4 and exhale for a count of 8. Repeat this four times, deepening your inhale and exhale with each breath. Now close your eyes and begin to imagine what your best health looks like. What does it sound, feel, smell, look and taste like? Really see it from the big picture down to the smallest detail. The first question you may want to ask yourself is: what is your motivation for improving your health? Explore that: how would your life be different if this were to happen? Would improving your health impact other areas of your life? What might those be? If your health improved, what is the first thing you would do? How would this make you feel? With whom would you be spending your time? How would you be spending your time?

So what do you think? What did you see? How did that feel? I know I am asking a lot of questions. Don't let them overwhelm you. If you didn't see anything this time, it's okay. You have to give yourself permission to trust the process. It will come, I promise. If you did see your vision, take note of what excited you, surprised you and provided comfort. Build on it and nourish it.

The first time a mentor led me through this type of visualization and I truly allowed myself to indulge my senses and embrace that I was creating my future, I felt **weightless**. I felt **liberated**. My mood shifted and I was **elated**. The heaviness I had felt pushing down on my shoulders disappeared. Even my kids noticed that something was different. This sensation lasted all day. It felt magical. I now make it a habit to visualize what I want to create for myself each morning so that my intention is set and my goal-achieving machine of a brain knows what it needs to do.

I invite you to imagine your ideal vision for each facet of your life. You may want to focus on just one area at a time so it doesn't feel overwhelming. You can repeat the line of questioning used above for every aspect of your life that you ranked less than a 10.

Now that you are well on your way to visualizing your "perfect 10" and can "see" how amazing it will look, feel, taste, sound and smell when it is realized, you can create it. You may not know exactly how or when yet, but that's okay. Trust that your brain is working for you to achieve your goal. As long as you trust your gut, you will be successful.

Swift Skin Action
Start creating the life you crave and live it! Get these worksheets as printables.

www.drskinwhisperer.com

Chapter 8:
SELF-CARE IS NOT SELFISH

"Love and compassion are necessities, not luxuries. Without them, humanity cannot survive"

Dalai Lama

As a physician, a mom and a spouse, I always felt like there was no good time to take a time-out. Each day felt like a never-ending cycle of rushing around from one thing to the next: work, kids' activities, laundry, grocery shopping, more kids' activities, meetings, eat, sleep, and repeat. I put exercise in the mix as an endurance runner, but I will be honest with you, the hours spent running and training were not truly done from a place of love for myself or my body. I did it out of obligation. I felt like I had to push myself beyond my limits, despite chronic pain, as a way to mold my appearance to be "pleasing" to societal norms. My childhood wounds from being teased for what was on my skin had transcended to how I viewed my appearance overall and I was in search of acceptance and gratification. The stories I had crafted for myself of not feeling "enough" had woven themselves into so many areas of my life. There was a feeling of not being smart enough, successful enough, thin enough, likable enough. Despite having an abundance of love from my family, a great career and the ability to provide for all my needs, I felt something was missing.

Until I discovered that spot on my arm and my worst nightmare became my reality, I was deafened by the incessant chatter in my mind. I had been unable to hear what my heart was trying to ask for, those challenging and often paralyzing questions like: *Who are you being? What is it you truly want? What do you need to do next to make it your new reality?* Being diagnosed with skin cancer, followed by a series of other health issues that piled on in the months following, was the catalyst for me to shut off the chatter. In those moments, I realized that I had to take care of my "self."

Does the idea of self-care feel selfish, self-indulgent, and insignificant? I get it, believe me. Clearly, I ignored the importance of this concept for most of my life. But what I learned through my journey is that self-care is the exact opposite of selfish. It is a vital form of self-acceptance, self-love and self-preservation. It's a necessity, not an indulgence. Caring for yourself is the foundation for positive and healthy relationships with others. Without a commitment to care for yourself, the effort of caring for others can become shrouded in emotional exhaustion, resentment and malcontent. Take it from me, I've been there and it's not pretty. Taking time to care for yourself empowers you to become resilient in the face of the curveballs life throws your way. And let's be honest, there's no shortage of those.

As you have gone on this journey with me throughout these pages, you have taken notice and learned how to nourish your skin, body and mind. The next step is to nurture your observations, make new decisions, implement the new habits you've been developing and reinforce the healthy habits you have already established. So how do you nurture yourself to ensure your success? I've found the following ideas effective, efficient and invaluable when it comes to nurturing the "self."

NEGOTIATE YOUR NON-NEGOTIABLES

What is really important to you? Have you truly figured out what matters to you most? If the sh*t hit the fan tomorrow, would you hesitate making decisions because you don't have a clear vision of what ultimately guides you in your life? As we have touched on, clarity is your key to feeling empowered and in control. These are what I call your non-negotiables.

Non-negotiables are the items, experiences, people or places that make your heart happy. They feed your soul. Nourishment is for your entire being, not just your belly and your skin. Rooted in your principles and values, non-negotiables define not only what you will and won't accept from others, but also what you will and won't accept from yourself.

Non-negotiables can be anything: weekly date nights, scheduling daily exercise, 10pm bedtime, picking your kids up from school, work-free weekends. When you clearly define what is important to you and you are prepared to follow through no matter what, you're stepping into your power.

Ready to define your non-negotiables? Here is a simple formula:

Get specific: Brainstorm what matters to you most. Differentiate your "nice to haves" from your "must haves." Write down your "must haves." These define what truly matters to you.

Get aligned: Do your non-negotiables align with your values and your goals? If not, go back to the previous point and get specific again.

Get selective: By adding in more of what aligns with your true passions, you will naturally crowd out the relationships and obligations that no longer serve your health or happiness. Think about those three to five people I asked you about in the last chapter. Do you want them to stay in your life or do they need to go? This is probably one of the hardest questions to answer and I acknowledge this. I am asking because your heart could be whispering or even shouting at you to take action, yet out of obligation, fear, worry or a million other reasons, you can't hear it. This is my loving attempt to be a megaphone for your emotional wellbeing.

Get talking: With your non-negotiables defined, share them with the most important people in your world: family, friends, co-workers. Communicating what matters most to you reinforces your intentions.

PRACTICE GRATITUDE

First of all I want to thank **you** for spending your time with me while you read these pages. I am honored to have this opportunity to share this book with you. Most importantly, I invite you to acknowledge yourself and give thanks for how amazing you are. Seriously, you **are** amazing! Just as you are, right here, right now. You are taking time to pay attention to what you see and who you are being in your skin so you can live as the best version of yourself. That is a big deal! Celebrate it!

There are so many reasons why cultivating a gratitude practice can nurture your sense of "self." The following are scientifically proven benefits for giving thanks:

Stress buster: Gratitude can pull you out of a negative mindset and put things into perspective. With the havoc stress inflicts on your skin and literally shaving years off our life, giving thanks packs a powerful punch.

Fewer aches and pains: Grateful people take care of their health, exercise more and experience greater longevity.

Better sleep: Practicing gratitude before bed can help you sleep better and longer.

Mental strength: Gratitude not only alleviates stress but contributes to fostering resilience and overcoming trauma.

Boosts self-esteem: I cannot stress enough that self-esteem is an essential component to optimal performance in all areas of your life and giving thanks amplifies your efforts. Gratitude helps kick comparison and resentment to the curb when you appreciate all that you do have.

Strengthens relationships: Expressing gratitude can improve relationships and facilitate communication to work through problems or concerns.

Amps up optimism: Gratitude both helps you think more positively and helps others feel more positively towards you. Better yet, the more you think about what you are grateful for, the more you discover to be grateful.

Whichever way you choose to practice gratitude, whether it be keeping a journal, jotting it down on scrap paper or verbalizing it to yourself or to others, practicing it consistently will do your "self" good.

BE MINDFUL

Taking notice — being conscious or aware of something — is the underpinning of mindfulness, so whether you realized it or not during your journey throughout these pages, you have been cultivating your mindfulness practice. As Thich Nhat Hahn shares, "Mindfulness gives you the inner space and quietness that allows you to look deeply, to find out who you are and what you want to do with your life."

Bringing your attention to the "right now" and being in this moment is one of the keys to creating the life you crave and living it, because your present is your future in the making. Through the practice of focusing on where you are now and tapping into your senses — what you see, hear, taste, feel and touch — you raise your awareness of sensations that you may wish to hold onto and cherish, as well as those you may want to let go. It also opens the door to the possibility of creating new sensations — ones you welcome.

Here is an exercise I have found incredibly valuable for nurturing a practice of mindfulness on a daily basis that you can do in less than 5 minutes.

To get started, find a comfortable chair where your back can be supported and your head is free to move. It doesn't require complete silence, though to maximize your benefit, it's beneficial to shut off digital notifications and silence your cell phone to minimize your distractions.

First, close your eyes and take notice of your breathing. Is it fast, slow, shallow or deep? The quickest way to shift your energy is to change the way you are breathing. Begin by breathing in for a count of 4 and breathing out for a count of 4. Repeat this for a few cycles. As you feel comfortable, you can breathe in for a count of 4 and extend your exhale to a count of 6 and then to a count of 8. Take at least 10 breaths like this to help you switch into your relaxation state.

Second, all you are going to be doing is taking notice of your senses. Without judgement, you are merely tuning in to your body and your environment. Begin with sight. See what you are **seeing** behind your closed lids. Is it totally dark or do you see light dancing on your cell membranes? Next hear what you are **hearing** from the loudest sound to the most subtle. Feel what you are **feeling**, from the air circulating in your nostrils, to the clothing on your skin, to where your body meets the chair. Are there areas of tension, discomfort or euphoria? What smells are you **smelling**? Perhaps you don't smell anything and that is okay. Finally, taste what you are **tasting**. Often there is a lingering taste in our mouths from toothpaste, food or it could be the absence of taste that gets your attention.

Now that you have become aware of your senses from top to bottom individually, layer them on top of one another and take a few final breaths. Gently and slowly open your eyes.

In a few short minutes, you will feel relaxed and more connected to yourself and your environment. That's what you're aiming for anyway. If it feels awkward or uncomfortable at the beginning, know that this is a totally normal feeling. They call it a practice for a reason. There is no such thing as perfection. It is the consistency of practice where you reap the benefits.

MEDITATE

By raising your awareness and bringing your focus to the present moment, I like to think of mindfulness as the appetizer to your meditation practice. Meditation moves beyond noticing and gives you permission to let it all go. As you become aware of your senses, there may be thoughts filtering into your consciousness that you interpret as distractions. It's okay. Your mind does not have to be quiet. In fact, it shouldn't be. Your thoughts are as automatic as your heart beating, so if you stop thinking, you've stopped living. You're in the midst of creating an amazing life right now, so just let your brain do its thing. Acknowledge whatever it is, then give yourself permission to let it go. Come back to your breath and the present moment.

Studies have shown that meditation can reduce your level of stress, boost your immunity and heart health and improve your concentration. The most important benefit of meditation from my perspective is increased self-awareness and self-acceptance. Meditation teaches you about your emotions and how to become more detached from them. An emotion, thought or sensation is something that you have, but it does not define who you are.

MOVE YOUR BODY

The benefits of exercise are well established: from decreasing your blood pressure, to losing weight, increasing energy, boosting immunity and decreasing your stress levels. But here's the most important thing I want to impart: Move your body with the intention of loving on it and your "self" rather than out of punishment for not feeling like "enough." Moving your body is not about "getting abs" or carving out a sexy tush, though these may be bonus by-products. Exercise is about getting stronger, building endurance and nourishing your muscles, tendons and bones so that your body can function at its optimal capacity and support you in accomplishing whatever you want to do with minimal if any limitations.

As I shared, I was an endurance runner, running marathons and ultra-marathons. As much as I enjoyed the camaraderie of my running gals, my desire to run was fueled by a compulsion to fill my void of not feeling "enough." I literally ran myself to the ground. During a training run, I felt the most excruciating pain I have ever felt and it dropped me to my knees. I had to crawl to a signpost to get back on my feet. It turns out I had torn my hip and had to undergo reconstructive surgery to repair it. From being incredibly active, I was forced to be incredibly still as I recovered from my injury.

This was an important lesson for me that I want to pass on to you: Too much of a good thing is not always a good thing. While moderate exercise reaps big benefits, intense exercise, especially endurance sports, can put a significant amount of stress on your body. Studies have shown that endurance running in particular can cause cortisol levels to soar, which triggers inflammation. And we know well by now the toll inflammation takes on your body and your skin.

Exercise can take many shapes and forms. From raking leaves to chasing after your kids, going for a walk in nature, a good romp in bed, having a dance party in your living room or taking a yoga, pilates or high intensity interval training class, all of it can boost your mood and your health. Whatever you choose, show yourself some love by moving in a way that feels good for your body and your mind.

CLEAN HOUSE

The foundation for living as the healthiest and happiest version of yourself rests upon removing obstacles that are standing in the way of your wellness. What obstacles am I talking about? Clutter. Physical clutter. Mental clutter. Emotional clutter. We all have a lot of stuff that fills our homes, our minds, our daily lives.

Stuff that we don't need. Don't use. Don't want. Stuff that isn't serving us in a positive way. Think of living without clutter as one of your non-negotiables.

One of the best ways to nurture the success of your journey is to clean your house and make room for life's important things… which actually aren't things at all.

Ready to declutter?

Simple declutter formula

1. Sell, donate or recycle the stuff that no longer brings you joy. Get rid of everything you are keeping out of obligation or the myth that "someday" it will fit or get used.

2. Hold onto everything that fills your heart with happiness. Ditch the rest. This applies to everything, including people in your life that suck your energy rather than fuel it. You deserve an upgrade in every aspect of your life. Don't forget that.

3. Make room for more: more passion, more experiences, more freedom, more contentment. Remember, it's your time to be selective. Add in what aligns with your true passions, as this will naturally crowd out the relationships and obligations that no longer serve your health or happiness. I know it can sometimes be hard to get started, but I promise you, it's worth it.

4. When in doubt, just breathe. Deeply, slowly and completely. Take your time, take time out, take a bath, read a book, go for a walk, and most importantly be kind and patient with yourself.

By joining me in this journey of noticing, nourishing and nurturing yourself from the outside in and the inside out, you are an integral part of revolutionizing the delivery of skincare. I believe you deserve to feel confident and comfortable in your skin and I know that experience is possible for you. You've got this and I've got your back!

Remember, it's not about perfection; it's about consistency. Life presents its challenges, and although we may not get to choose the hand we're dealt, we can choose how we play it. Finding ways to reframe your responses to any given challenge is one your best anti-aging strategies. With that in mind, here's a checklist to help you nurture your new habits starting today.

1. ***Meditation and mindfulness:*** Living in the moment and letting go of feelings about past events will serve you well. Consider guided meditations offered online, like with Hay House (search on iTunes), or just close your eyes, focus on your breath and let your stress melt away.

2. ***Find your people:*** Surround yourself with people who support you and your interests. Those are your people. Lose the people who bring you down.

3. ***Get outside:*** Breathe in the fresh air and connect with nature. By changing your scenery, you can change your perspective.

4. ***Move your body:*** It doesn't have to be an intense workout, although those can feel great too! Just move. Turn on some music, have your own personal dance party or go for a walk. When all your focus is on your movement, it's amazingly cleansing for the mind!

5. ***Eat well:*** Good nutrition is critical in providing the building blocks necessary to make neurotransmitters like serotonin and dopamine, which help elevate your mood and alleviate stress.

6. ***Be true to yourself:*** What brings you joy? Focus on that. By adding in things that align with your true passions, they will naturally crowd out the relationships and obligations that no longer serve your health or happiness.

To your longevity and health!

Chapter 9:
FINAL THOUGHTS

"When you want something, all the universe conspires in helping you achieve it."

Paulo Coelho

You have the power to look younger, radiate beauty, create and live the life you crave starting now! You have all the tools and all the resources to make it happen. And you have a process that will guide you step by step through everything you need to do. You can read this guide over and over again.

This is a journey. You can set the pace that feels **right for you**. In time, if you follow these steps, you can experience increased energy and youthfulness as you nourish your body with the nutrients it needs and protect yourself from the elements that age you. Your beauty will radiate because you are nourishing yourself on all levels. By making yourself a priority, you become more aligned with what matters most to you. I have been on this journey myself and I am here to support you on yours. There's no reason why you can't do it too. You are not alone.

HERE IS MY VISION FOR YOU

This is your time! It's your time to start hearing what your skin is telling you about what your body needs to thrive. It's your time to acknowledge yourself for the amazing being you are right now. It's your time to notice, nourish and nurture your skin, body and mind so you can live life on your terms, not someone else's. You deserve radiant health and emotional wellbeing.

I want to thank you for having the clarity and confidence to invest in yourself, invest in this book and to trust me as you embark on this journey. I am here to invest in you. I want to support and celebrate you, and more than anything, I want you to be successful.

If you love what you've read, I would absolutely love to hear from you, get to know you better and learn how I can further support you... *And* if you did enjoy this book, please leave a review on Amazon, it would mean the world to me.

Visit my website: www.drkeirabarr.com.

And follow me on social media.

- LinkedIn: https://www.linkedin.com/in/keirabarr/
- Instagram: https://www.instagram.com/resiliencyblueprint/
- Facebook: https://www.facebook.com/resiliencyblueprint

With big love and gratitude,

Dr. Keira

REFERENCES

Chapter 2.

1. Burke KE. Photoaging: the role of oxidative stress. G Ital Dermatol Venereol.2010;145(4):445-459
2. Greenlee H, Gammon MD, Abrahamson PE, et al. Prevalence and predictors of antioxidant supplement use during breast cancer treatment: the Long Island Breast Cancer Study Project. Cancer.2009;115(14):3271-3282
3. Huang CC, Hsu BY, Wu NL, et al. Anti-photoaging effects of soy isoflavone extract (aglycone and acetylglucoside form) from soybean cake. Int J Mol Sci.2010;11(12):4782-4795
4. Ji C, Yang B, Yang Z, et al. Ultra-violet B (UVB)-induced skin cell death occurs through a cyclophilin D intrinsic signaling pathway. Biochem Biophys Res Commun.2012;425(4):825-829
5. Kovacic P, Somanathan R. Dermal toxicity and environmental contamination: electron transfer, reactive oxygen species, oxidative stress, cell signaling, and protection by antioxidants. Rev Environ Contam Toxicol.2010;203:119-138
6. Lademann J, Vergou T, Darvin ME, et al. Influence of Topical, Systemic and Combined Application of Antioxidants on the Barrier Properties of the Human Skin. Skin Pharmacol Physiol.2016;29(1):41-46
7. Lademann J, Schanzer S, Meinke M, et al. Interaction between carotenoids and free radicals in human skin. Skin Pharmacol Physiol.2011;24(5):238-244

8. Magnani ND, Muresan XM, Belmonte G, et al. Skin Damage Mechanisms Related to Airborne Particulate Matter Exposure. Toxicol Sci.2016;149(1):227-236
9. Marchiani A, Rozzo C, Fadda A, et al. Curcumin and curcumin-like molecules: from spice to drugs. Curr Med Chem.2014;21(2):204-222
10. Mizutani T, Masaki H. Anti-photoaging capability of antioxidant extract from Camellia japonica leaf. Exp Dermatol.2014;23 Suppl 1:23-26
11. Murr C, Schroecksnadel K, Winkler C, et al. Antioxidants may increase the probability of developing allergic diseases and asthma. Med Hypotheses.2005;64(5):973-977
12. Padayatty SJ, Katz A, Wang Y, et al. Vitamin C as an antioxidant: evaluation of its role in disease prevention. J Am Coll Nutr.2003;22(1):18-35
13. Pillai S, Oresajo C, Hayward J. Ultraviolet radiation and skin aging: roles of reactive oxygen species, inflammation and protease activation, and strategies for prevention of inflammation-induced matrix degradation — a review. Int J Cosmet Sci.2005;27(1):17-34
14. Trueb RM. Association between smoking and hair loss: another opportunity for health education against smoking? Dermatology.2003;206(3):189-191
15. Soeur J, Eilstein J, Lereaux G, et al. Skin resistance to oxidative stress induced by resveratrol: from Nrf2 activation to GSH biosynthesis. Free Radic Biol Med.2015;78:213-223; PMID: 25451641.
16. Wang Y, Zhao L, Wang D, et al. Anthocyanin-rich extracts from blackberry, wild blueberry, strawberry, and chokeberry: antioxidant activity and inhibitory effect on oleic acid-induced hepatic steatosis in vitro. J Sci Food Agric.2016;96(7):2494-2503

Chapter 3.

1. Agin PP. Water resistance and extended wear sunscreens. Dermatol Clin. 2006;24(10):75–79
2. American Academy of Dermatology. Facts about sunscreen.
3. Autier P, Boniol M, Doré JF. Sunscreen use and increased duration of intentional sun exposure: still a burning issue. Int J Cancer. 2007;121(1):1–5

4. Bech-Thomsen N, Wulf HC. Sunbathers' application of sunscreen is probably inadequate to obtain the sun protection factor assigned to the preparation. Photodermatol Photoimmunol Photomed. 1992–1993;9(6):242–244

5. Bulliard JL. Site-specific risk of cutaneous malignant melanoma and pattern of sun exposure in New Zealand. Int J Cancer. 2000;85(5):627–632

6. Butler ST, Fosko SW. Increased prevalence of left-sided skin cancers. J Am Acad Dermatol. 2010;63(6):1006–1010

7. Cesarini JP, Chardon A, Binet O, Hourseau C, Grollier JF. High-protection sunscreen formulation prevents UVB-induced sunburn cell formation. Photodermatol. 1989;6(1):20–23

8. Dal H, Boldemann C, Lindelof B. Does relative melanoma distribution by body site 1960–2004 reflect changes in intermittent exposure and intentional tanning in the Swedish population? Eur J Dermatol. 2007;17(5):428–434

9. De Gruijl FR. Skin cancer and solar UV radiation. Eur J Cancer. 1999;35(14):2003–2009

10. De Laat A, van der Leun JC, de Gruikl FR. Carcinogenesis induced by UVA (365-nm) radiation: the dose-time dependence of tumor formation in hairless mice. Carcinogenesis. 1997;18(5):1013–1020

11. Diffey B. Sunscreens: expectation and realization. Photodermatol Photoimmunol Photomed. 2009;25(5):233–236

12. Draelos ZD. Compliance and sunscreens. Dermatol Clin. 2006;24(1):101–104

13. Dummer R, Maier T. UV protection and skin cancer. Recent Results Cancer Res. 2002;160:7–12

14. Eide MJ, Weinstock MA. Public health challenges in sun protection. Dermatol Clin. 2006;24(1):119–124

15. Filipe P, Silva JN, Silva R,. Stratum corneum is an effective barrier to TiO2 and ZnO nanoparticle percutaneous absorption. Skin Pharmacol Physiol. 2009;22(5):266–275

16. Green A, Williams G, Neale R,. Daily sunscreen application and beta carotene supplementation in prevention of basal-cell and squamous-cell carcinomas of the skin: a randomised controlled trial. Lancet. 1999;354(9180):723–729

17. Green AC, Williams GM, Logan V, Strutton GM. Reduced melanoma after regular sunscreen use: randomized trial follow-up. J Clin Oncol. 2010;29(3):257–263
18. Green AC, Williams GM. Point: sunscreen use is a safe and effective approach to skin cancer prevention. Cancer Epidemiol Biomarkers Prev. 2007 Oct;16(10):1921-2.
19. Han J, Colditz GA, Hunter DJ. Risk factors for skin cancers: a nested case-control study with the Nurses' Health Study. Int J Epidemiol. 2006;35(6):1514–1521
20. Hexsel CL, Bangert SD, Herbert AA, Lim HW. Current sunscreen issues: 2007 Food and Drug Administration sunscreen labeling recommendations and combination sunscreen/insect repellent products. J Am Acad Dermatol. 2008;59(2):316–323
21. Holick MF. The cutaneous photosynthesis of previtamin D3: a unique photoendocrine system. J Invest Dermatol. 1981;77(1):51–58
22. Holick MF. Sunlight, UV-radiation, vitamin D and skin cancer: how much sunlight do we need? Adv Exp Med Biol. 2008;624:1–15
23. Huncharek M, Kupelnick B. Use of topical sunscreens and the risk of malignant melanoma: a meta-analysis of 9067 patients from 11 case-control studies. Am J Public Health. 2002;92(7):1173–1177
24. Janjua NR, Mogensen B, Andersson AM,. Systemic absorption of the sunscreens benzophenone-3, octyl-methoxycinnamate, and 3-(4-methyl-benzylidene) camphor after whole-body topical application and reproductive hormone levels in humans. J Invest Dermatol. 2004;123(10):57–61
25. Kechichian E, Ezzedine K. Vitamin D and the Skin: An Update for Dermatologists. Am J Clin Dermatol. 2017 Oct 9.
26. Kimlin M, Harrison S, Nowak M, Moore M, Brodie A, Lang C. Does a high UV environment ensure adequate vitamin D status? J Photochem Photobiol B. 2007;89(2–3):139–147
27. Kricker A, Armstrong BK, English DR, Heenan PJ. Does intermittent sun exposure cause basal cell carcinoma? A case control study in Western Australia. Int J Cancer. 1995;60(4):489–494

28. Lin JS, Eder M, Weinmann S. Behavioral counseling to prevent skin cancer: a systematic review form the U.S. Preventive Services Task Force. Ann Intern Med. 2011;154:190–201
29. Lowe NJ. Photoprotection. Semin Dermatol. 1990;9(1):78–83
30. Marrot L, Meunier JR. Skin DNA photodamage and its biologic consequences. J Am Acad Dermatol. 2008;58(5 suppl 2):S139–S148
31. Marks R, Foley PA, Jolley D, Knight KR, Harrison J, Thompson SC. The effect of regular sunscreen use on vitamin D levels in an Australian population. Arch Dermatol. 1995;131(4):415–421
32. Matsuoka LY, Ide L, Wortsman J, MacLaughlin JA, Holick MF. Sunscreens suppress cutaneous vitamin D3 synthesis. J Clin Endocrinol Metab. 1987;64(6):1165–1168
33. Menzies SW. Is sun exposure a major cause of melanoma? Yes. BJM. 2009;337:a763
34. McKenzie RL, Bjorn LO, Bais A, Lyasad M. Changes in biologically active ultraviolet radiation reaching the Earth's surface. Photochem Photobiol Sci. 2003;2(1):5–15
35. Nash JF. Human safety and efficacy of ultraviolet filters and sunscreen products. Dermatol Clin. 2006;24(1):35–51
36. Naylor MF, Boyd A, Smith DW,. High sun protection factor sunscreens in the suppression of actinic neoplasia. Arch Dermatol. 1995;131(2):170–175
37. Nohynek GJ, Antignanc E, Re T, Toutain H. Safety assessment of personal care products/cosmetics and their ingredients. Toxicol Appl Pharmacol. 2010;243(2):239–259
38. Norval M, Wulf HC. Does chronic sunscreen use reduce vitamin D production to insufficient levels? Br J Dermatol. 2009;161(4):732–736
39. Oberyszyn TM. Non-melanoma skin cancer: importance of gender, immunosuppressive status and vitamin D. Cancer Lett. 2008;261(2):127–136
40. Osterwalder U, Herzog B. Sun protection factors: worldwide confusion. Br J Dermatol. 2009;161(suppl 2):13–24
41. Palm MD, O'Donoghue MN. Update on photoprotection. Dermatol Ther. 2007;20(5):360–376

42. Pfahlberg A, Kolmel KF, Gefeller O; Febim Study Group. Timing of excessive ultraviolet radiation and melanoma: epidemiology does not support the existence of a critical period of high susceptibility to solar ultraviolet radiation-induced melanoma. Br J Dermatol. 2001;144(3):471–475
43. Reichrath J, Saternus R, Vogt T. Endocrine actions of vitamin D in skin: Relevance for photocarcinogenesis of non-melanoma skin cancer, and beyond. Mol Cell Endocrinol. 2017 Sep 15;453:96-102.
44. Ridley AJ, Whiteside JR, McMillan TJ, Allison SL. Cellular and sub-cellular responses to UVA in relation to carcinogenesis. Int J Radiat Biol. 2009;85(3):177–195
45. Rigel DS. Cutaneous ultraviolet exposure and its relationship to the development of skin cancer. J Am Acad Dermatol. 2008;58:S129–S132
46. Rigel DS, Rigel EG, Rigel AC. Effects of altitude and latitude on ambient UVB radiation. J Am Acad Dermatol. 1999;40(1):114–116
47. Rosso S, Zanetti R, Martinez C,. The multicentre south European study 'Helios'. II: Different sun exposure patterns in the aetiology of basal cell and squamous cell carcinomas of the skin. Br J Cancer. 1996;73(11):1447–1454
48. Russak JE, Chen T, Appa Y, Rigel DS. A comparison of sunburn protection of high-sun protection factor (SPF) sunscreens: SPF 85 sunscreen is significantly more protective than SPF 50. J Am Acad Dermatol. 2010;62(2):348–349
49. Sambandan DR, Ratner D. Sunscreens: an overview and update. JAAD. 2011;64(4):749–758
50. Scott JF, Das LM, Ahsanuddin S, Qiu Y, Binko AM, Traylor ZP et al. Oral Vitamin D Rapidly Attenuates Inflammation from Sunburn: An Interventional Study. J Invest Dermatol 2017 Oct;137(10):2078-2086
51. Schaefer H, Redelmaier TE, eds. Skin Barrier: Principles of Percutaneous Absorption. Basel, Switerland: Karger AG; 1996:118–128, 191–193
52. Schlumpf M, Cotton B, Conscience M. In vitro and in vivo estrogenicity of UV screens. Environ Health Perspect. 2001;109(3):239–244
53. Sehedic D, Hardy-Boismartel A, Conuteau C, Coiffard LJ. Are cosmetic products which include an SPF appropriate for daily use? Arch Dermatol Res. 2009;301(8):603–608

54. Seite S, Colige A, Piquemal-Vivenot P,. A full-UV spectrum absorbing daily use cream protects human skin against biological changes occurring in photoaging. Photodermatol Photoimmunol Photomed. 2000;16(4):147–155
55. Seité S, Fourtanier AM. The benefits of daily photoprotection. J Am Acad Dermatol. 2008;58(5 suppl 2):S160–S166
56. Sjerobabski Masnec I, Poduje S. Photoaging. Coll Antropol. 2008;32(suppl 2):177–180
57. Skin Cancer Foundation. www.skincancer.org
58. Slominski AT, Brożyna AA, Skobowiat C, Zmijewski MA, Kim TK, Janjetovic Z et al. On the role of classical and novel forms of vitamin D in melanoma progression and management. J Steroid Biochem Mol Biol. 2017.
59. Stechschulte S, Kirsner R, Federman D. Sunscreens for Non-Dermatologists: What you Should Know when Counseling Patients. Postgraduate Medicine Vol. 123; 4, 2011
60. Sollitto RB, Kraemer KH, DiGiovanna JJ. Normal vitamin D levels can be maintained despite rigorous photoprotection: six years' experience with xeroderma pigmentosum. J Am Acad Dermatol. 1997;37(6):942–947 Stern ST, McNeil SE. Nanotechnology safety concerns revisited. Toxicol Sci. 2008;101(1):4–21
61. Stern RS, Weinstein MC, Baker SG. Risk reduction for nonmelanoma skin cancer with childhood sunscreen use. Arch Dermatol. 1986;122(5):537–545
62. Sunscreen drug products for over-the-counter human use. Proposed amendment of final monograph. Proposed rule, Federal Register. Monday, August 27, 2007;72(165):49070–49122
63. Tanner PR. Sunscreen product formulation. Dermatol Clin. 2006;24(1):53–62
64. Vainio H, Miller AB, Bianchini F. An international evaluation of the cancer-preventive potential of sunscreens. Int J Cancer. 2000;88(5):838–842
65. Van de Pols JC, Williams GM, Pandeya N, Logan V, Green AC. Prolonged prevention of squamous cell carcinoma of the skin by regular sunscreen use. Cancer Epidemiol Biomarkers Prev. 2006;15(12):2546–2548

66. Walter SD, King WD, Marrett LD. Association of cutaneous malignant melanoma with intermittent exposure to ultraviolet radiation: results of a case-control study in Ontario, Canada. Int J Epidemiol. 1999;28(3):418–427

67. Wang SQ, Dusza SW. Assessment of sunscreen knowledge: a pilot survey. Br J Dermatol. 2009;161(suppl 3):28–32

68. Wlaschek M, Tantcheva-Poor I, Naderi L,. Solar UV irradiation and dermal photoaging. J Photochem Photobiol B. 2001;63(1–3):41–51

69. Wulf H, Stender I, Lock-Andersen J. Sunscreens used at the beach do not protect against erythema: a new definition of SPF is proposed. Photodermatol Photoimmunol Photomed. 1997;13(4):129–132

70. Young AR. Acute effects of UVR on human eyes and skin. Prog Biophys Mol Biol. 2006;92(1):80–85

Chapter 4.

1. Andréasson K, Alrawi Z, Persson A, et al. Intestinal dysbiosis is common in systemic sclerosis and associated with gastrointestinal and extraintestinal features of disease. Arthritis Res Ther.2016;18(1):278;

2. Accorsi-Neto A, et al. Effects of isoflavones on the skin of postmenopausal women: a pilot study. Clinics (Sao Paulo) 2009;64(6):505-10.

3. A Jain, C Manghani, S Kohli, D Nigam and V Rani. Tea and human health: dark shadows. Toxicology Letters, vol 220, no1, p82-87, 2013.

4. AL Chen, CH Hsu, JK Lin et al. Phase I clinical trial of curcumin, a chemopreventative agent, in patients with high risk or premalignant lesions. Anticancer Research, vol 21, no4, p2895-2900, 2001.Asgari MM, Chren M-M, Warton EM, Friedman GD, White E. Supplement Use and Risk of Cutaneous Squamous Cell Carcinoma. Journal of the American Academy of Dermatology. 2011;65(6):1145-1151.

5. Caini S, Cattaruzza S, Bendinelli B, Tosti G, Masala G, Gnagnarella P, Assedi M, Stanganelli I, Palli D, Gandini S. Coffee, tea and caffeine intake and the risk of non-melanoma skin cancer: a review of the literature and meta-analysis. Eur J Nutr. 2017 Feb;56(1):1-12

6. David L. Maurice C, Carmody R, Gootenberg D, Button J, Wolfe D et al. Diet rapidly and reproducibly alters the human gut microbiome. Nature 505, 559–563 (23 January 2014)

7. Damian, D. L. (2017), Nicotinamide for skin cancer chemoprevention. Australas J Dermatol, 58: 174–180
8. DR Bickers, M athar. Novel approaches to chemoprevention of skin cancer. Journal of Dermatology vol27, no11, p691-695.2000
9. Fortes et al. A protective effect of the Mediterranean diet for cutaneous melanoma. Int J Epidemiology; 2008: 37(5):1018-29M Singh, S Suman and Y Shulka. New Enlightenment of Skin Cancer Chemoprevention through Phytochemicals: In Vitro and In Vivo Studies and the Underlying Mechanisms. BioMed Research International vol 2014
10. Hakimzadeh H, Ghazanfari T, Rahmati B, Naderimanesh H. Cytotoxic effect of garlic extract and its fractions on Sk-mel3 melanoma cell line. Immunopharmacol Immunotoxicol. 2010;32:371–5
11. Harris RE, et al. Inverse association of non-steroidal anti-inflammatory drugs and malignant melanoma among women. Oncol Rep 2001;8(3):655-7.
12. Huang MT, et al. Inhibitory effects of curcumin on in vitro lipoxygenase and cyclooxygenase activities in mouse epidermis. Cancer Res 1991 51(3):813-9.Karimi G, Vahabzadeh M, Lari P, Rashedinia M, Moshiri M. "Silymarin", a Promising Pharmacological Agent for Treatment of Diseases. Iranian Journal of Basic Medical Sciences. 2011;14(4):308-317.
13. JK Kim, Y Kim, KM Na, YJ Surh, and TY Kim. [6]-gingerol prevents UVB-induced ROS production and COX-2 expression in vitro and in vivo. Free Radical Research, vol 41, no 5 p603-614, 2007.
14. Micek A, Godos J, Lafranconi A, Marranzano M, Pajak A.Caffeinated and decaffeinated coffee consumption and melanoma risk: a dose-response meta-analysis of prospective cohort studies. Int J Food Sci Nutr. 2017 Sep 11:1-10.M. Vaid, R Orasad, T Singh and S.K. Katiyar. Grape seed proanthocyanidins inhibit Melanoma cell invasiveness by reduction of pgE2 synthesis and reversal of Epithelial-to-Mesenchymal transition. PLoS ONE, vol 6
15. Minocha R, Damian DL, Halliday GM. Melanoma and nonmelanoma skin cancer chemoprevention: A role for nicotinamide?. Photodermatol Photoimmunol Photomed. 2017;00:1–8.ML Tsai, CS Lai, YH CHang, WJ Chen, T Ho, and MH Pan. Ptersostilben, a natural analogue of resveratrol potently inhibits 7,12-dimethylben[a]anthracene(DMBA/12O-tet-

radecanoylphorbol-13-acetate(TPA)induced mouse skin carcinogenesis. Food and Function, vol 3,no11,p1185-1194, 2012.

16. M Zaid, F Afaq, DN Syed, M Dreher, H Mukhtar. Inhibition of UVB mediated oxidative stress and markers of photoaging in immortalized HaCaT keratinocytes by pomegranate polyphenol extract POMx. Photochemistry and Photobiology, vol 83, no4 p882-888, 2007.

17. Nestor MS, Berman B, Swenson N. Safety and Efficacy of Oral Polypodium leucotomos Extract in Healthy Adult Subjects. The Journal of Clinical and Aesthetic Dermatology. 2015;8(2):19-23.

18. O'Neill CA, Monteleone G, McLaughlin JT, et al. The gut-skin axis in health and disease: A paradigm with therapeutic implications. Bioessays.2016;38(11):1167-1176

19. Owen RW, Giacosa A, Hull WE, Haubner R, Würtele G, Spiegelhalder B, Bartsch H. Olive-oil consumption and health: the possible role of antioxidants. Lancet Oncol. 2000 Oct;1:107-12.

20. Penta D, Somashekar BS, Meeran SM. Epigenetics of Skin Cancer: Interventions by selected bioactive Phytochemicals Photodermatol Photoimmunol Photomed. 2017 Oct

21. SK Katiyar, M Vaid, H van Steeg, and SM Meeran. Green tea polyphenols prevent uv induced immunosuppression by rapid repair of DNA damage and enhancement of nucleotide excision repair genes. Cancer Prevention Research, vol 3. No2 p179-189.2010.

22. Stoner GD, Mukhtar H. Polyphenols as cancer chemopreventive agents. J Cell Biochem Suppl. 1995; 22:169-80.

23. Toskes, P.P., 1993. Bacterial overgrowth of the gastrointestinal tract. Advances in Internal Medicine 38: 387-407.

24. ZY Wang, R Agarwal, DR Bickers, H Mukhtar. Protection against ultraviolet B radiation photocarcinogenesis in hairless mice by green tea polyphenols. Carcinogenesis, vol 12, no8, p1527-1530. 1991

25. Wells JM, Brummer RJ, Derrien M, et al. Homeostasis of the Gut Barrier and Potential Biomarkers. Am J Physiol Gastrointest Liver Physiol.2016

26. Williams S, Tamburic S, Lally C. Eating chocolate can significantly protect the skin from UV light. J Cosmet Dermatol.2009;8(3):169-173;

27. Wu S, et al. Citrus consumption and risk of basal cell carcinoma and squamous cell carcinoma of the skin. Carcinogenesis 2015;36:1162-1168.
28. Wu S, et al. Citrus consumption and risk of cutaneous malignant melanoma. J Clin Oncol 2015;33(23):2500-8.

Chapter 5.

1. Desotelle JA, Wilking MJ, Ahmad N. The Circadian Control of Skin and Cutaneous Photodamage. Photochemistry and photobiology. 2012;88(5):1037-1047
2. Esrefoglu M, Seyhan M, Gül M, Parlakpinar H, Batçioğlu K, Uyumlu B. Potent therapeutic effect of melatonin on aging skin in pinealectomized rats. J Pineal Res. 2005 Oct;39(3):231-7.
3. Goswami S, Haldar C. Melatonin as a possible antidote to UV radiation induced cutaneous damages and immune-suppression: An overview. J Photochem Photobiol B. 2015 Dec;153:281-8.
4. Greco M, Villani G, Mazzucchelli F, et al. Marked aging-related decline in efficiency of oxidative phosphorylation in human skin fibroblasts. FASEB J. 2003 Sep;17(12):1706-8.Gutierrez D, Arbesman J.Circadian Dysrhythmias, Physiological Aberrations, and the Link to Skin Cancer. Int J Mol Sci. 2016 Apr 26;17(5).
5. Markova-Car EP, Jurišić D, Ilić N, Kraljević Pavelić S. Running for time: circadian rhythms and melanoma. Tumour Biol. 2014 Sep;35(9):8359-68
6. Mazzaccoli G, Carughi S, De Cata A, La Viola M, Vendemiale G. Melatonin and cortisol serum levels in lung cancer patients at different stages of disease. Med Sci Monit. 2005;11:CR284–288
7. Scheuer C, Pommergaard HC, Rosenberg J, Gögenur I. Effect of topical application of melatonin cream 12.5% on cognitive parameters: A randomized, placebo-controlled, double-blind crossover study in healthy volunteers. J Dermatolog Treat. 2016 Nov;27(6):488-494.
8. Scheuer C, Pommergaard HC, Rosenberg J, Gögenur I. Melatonin's protective effect against UV radiation: a systematic review of clinical and experimental studies. Photodermatol Photoimmunol Photomed. 2014 Aug;30(4):180-8

9. Slominski AT, Zmijewski MA, Semak I, Kim TK, Janjetovic Z, Slominski RM, Zmijewski JW. Melatonin, mitochondria, and the skin. Cell Mol Life Sci. 2017 Nov;74(21):3913-3925.
10. Slominski A, Pisarchik A, Zbytek B, Tobin DJ, Kauser S, Wortsman J. Functional activity of serotoninergic and melatoninergic systems expressed in the skin. J Cell Physiol. 2003 Jul;196(1):144-53.
11. Slominski AT, Kleszczyński K, Semak I, Janjetovic Z, Zmijewski MA, Kim TK, Slominski RM, Reiter RJ, Fischer TW. Local melatoninergic system as the protector of skin integrity. Int J Mol Sci. 2014 Sep 30;15(10):17705-32.
12. Schernhammer ES, Hankinson SE. Urinary Melatonin Levels and Breast Cancer Risk. J Natl Cancer Inst. 2005;97:1084–1087.
13. Schernhammer ES, Berrino F, Krogh V, Secreto G, Micheli A, Venturelli E, Sieri S, Sempos CT, Cavalleri A, Schünemann HJ, Strano S, Muti P. Urinary 6-Sulfatoxymelatonin Levels and Risk of Breast Cancer in Postmenopausal Women. J Natl Cancer Inst. 2008;100:898–905.
14. Schernhammer ES, Hankinson SE. Urinary Melatonin Levels and Postmenopausal Breast Cancer Risk in the Nurses' Health Study Cohort. Cancer Epidemiol Biomarkers Prev. 2009;18:74–79.

Chapter 6.

1. Stokes, J.H. and Pillsbury, D.H., 1930. The effect on the skin of emotional and nervous states: theoretical and practical consideration of a gastrointestinal mechanism. Archives of Dermatology and Syphilology 22: 962-993.
2. Maltz, Maxwell. Psycho-Cybernetics: A New Way to Get More Living Out of Life. N. Hollywood, Calif: Wilshire Book, 1976.

Chapter 7.

1. Maltz, Maxwell. Psycho-Cybernetics: A New Way to Get More Living Out of Life. N. Hollywood, Calif: Wilshire Book, 1976.
2. Hanh, Thich Nhat. Silence: The Power of Quiet in a World Full of Noise. Harper Collins, 2015

Chapter 8.

1. Hanh, Thich Nhat. Silence: The Power of Quiet in a World Full of Noise. Harper Collins, 2015
2. McKeown, Greg. Essentialism: The Disciplined Pursuit of Less. First edition. Crown Business, 2014.

ABOUT THE AUTHOR

Dr. Keira L. Barr believes that everyone deserves to feel comfortable in their skin — and that the potential to do so exists inside each one of us. When we feel confident and comfortable in our skin, we make better choices in our lives. That's why Dr. Barr is dedicated to harnessing the power of self-awareness and self-confidence to transform the choices we make every day that impact our health, relationships and businesses.

Dr. Barr works to empower people, organizations and communities to nourish their skin and their minds as part of their journey towards resilient health. As an acclaimed global speaker, author, leader, and educator in her field, Dr. Barr is a cutting edge, dual board-certified dermatologist, who is known as an innovative thinker. She has shared her life-changing ideas in business, education, health and professional seminars on how to rejuvenate and amplify skin health naturally; reverse sun damage, prevent and manage skin cancer, and build confidence, self-awareness, self-esteem and resilience.

Dr. Barr shares her expertise as a domain subject matter expert, advisor to numerous start-ups, editor of multiple leading medical journals and researcher in ongoing clinical trials. As the Chief Wellness Officer of Resilient Health Institute (RHI), by embracing what is on the surface as well as what's below it, she is redefining the delivery of skincare.

Having authored numerous articles for professional and trade journals, and guest blogs, Dr. Barr has also been seen on PBS's *Ask Dr. Nandi*, as well as featured on podcasts, radio interviews and print media in all of the major metropolitan media markets.

She lives in the Pacific Northwest with her husband, two children and three dogs. With a lot of love and some creative juggling, there is never a dull moment.

Printed in Great Britain
by Amazon